協醫校刊

胡適題

Title-page of PUMC student yearbook THE UNISON 1931-1932.
Calligraphy of Dr. Hu Shih

CHINA
MEDICAL BOARD
AND
PEKING UNION
MEDICAL COLLEGE

A Chronicle of Fruitful Collaboration
1914-1951
BY
MARY E. FERGUSON

China Medical Board of New York, Inc.
NEW YORK
1970

 Peking Union Medical College Press

图书在版编目（CIP）数据

美国中华医学基金会与北京协和医学院：丰硕合作纪事：1914-1951 = China Medical Board and Peking Union Medical College. A Chronicle of Fruitful Collaboration (1914-1951)：英文 / (美) 福梅龄 (Mary E. Ferguson) 著. -- 北京：中国协和医科大学出版社, 2024. 8 (2024.9重印). -- ISBN 978-7-5679-2464-2

Ⅰ. D771.27；R199.2

中国国家版本馆CIP数据核字第2024L2Y053号

著作权合同登记：图字01-2024-3860 号

原著作者　福梅龄
责任编辑　李元君　白　兰
封面设计　邱晓俐
责任校对　张　麓
责任印制　黄艳霞
出版发行　中国协和医科大学出版社
　　　　　（北京市东城区东单三条9号　邮编100730　电话010-65260431）
网　　址　www.pumcp.com
印　　刷　北京联兴盛业印刷股份有限公司
开　　本　710mm×1000mm　　1/16
印　　张　19
字　　数　310千字
版　　次　2024年8月第1版
印　　次　2024年9月第2次印刷
定　　价　108.00元

（版权所有，侵权必究，如有印装质量问题，由本社发行部调换）

First China Medical Commission—1914

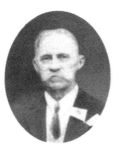

Dr. Harry Pratt Judson
Chairman

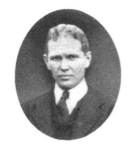

Dr. Francis W. Peabody

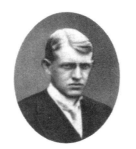

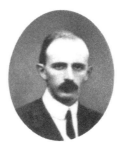

Mr. Roger S. Greene

Mr. George B. McKibbin
Secretary

Second China Medical Commission—1915

Left to right,
Dr. Wallace Buttrick
Chairman
Dr. F. T. Gates
Secretary
Dr. Simon Flexner
Mr. Roger S. Greene
Resident Director of CMB
Dr. William H. Welch

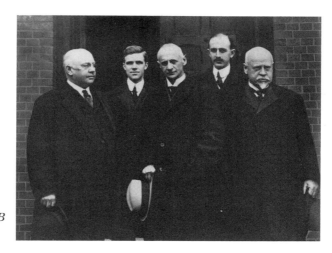

First Administrators

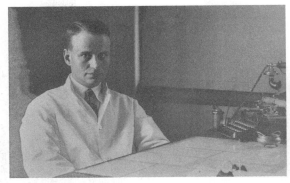

Dr. Franklin C. McLean
Director 1916-1920

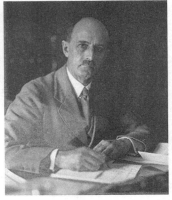

Mr. Roger S. Greene
Resident Director, CMB
1915-1933
Acting Director, PUMC
1929-1934

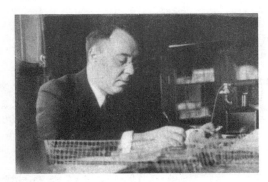

Dr. Richard M. Pearce
Acting Director 1920-1921

Dr. Henry S. Houghton
Director 1921-1928
Acting Director
1937-1946

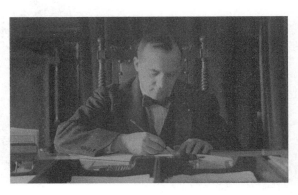

Laying the Cornerstone — September 24, 1917

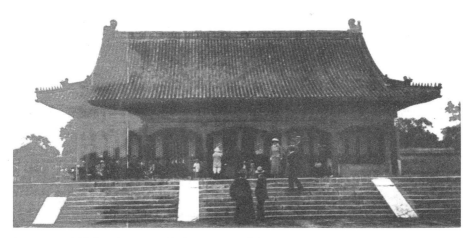

Ceremonial Hall of Prince Yu's Palace with US Marine Band on the terrace.

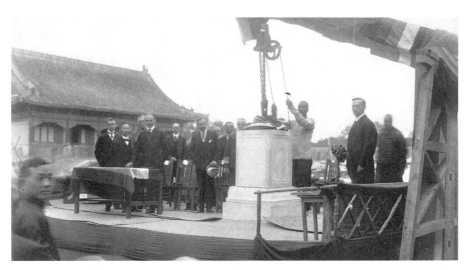

Left to right, Dr. McLean; Mr. Fan Yuan-lien, *Chinese Minister of Education*; Col. Frank S. Billings, *Chief of American Red Cross Commission to Russia*; Dr. Paul S. Reinsch, *American Minister to China*; Mr. Greene; Mr. Beilby Alston, *British Chargé d'Affaires*; *at extreme right*, Mr. Frank R. Bennett, in charge of CMB Architectural Office.

The Premedical School

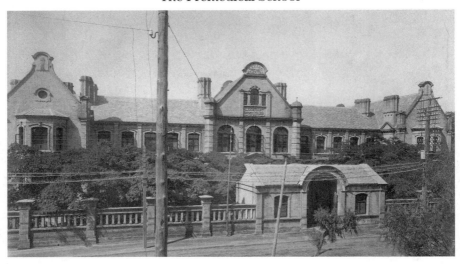

Lockhart Hall

FACULTY AND STAFF 1921-1922—*Left to right, front row:* Rev. Lorin Webster, Rev. C. H. Corbett, Dr. S. D. Wilson, Dr. Charles Packard, Mr. Ma Kiam; *second row:* Mr. B. R. Stephenson, Miss Emily Tilly, Miss Grace Huang, Miss Helen R. Downes, Mr. Aura E. Severinghaus, Mr. Yu I-fang, Mr. Frank M. Exner; *third row:* Mr. Leslie R. Severinghaus, Mr. N. K. Tang, Mr. E. C. Scott, Mr. C. M. Yu, Miss Edna Wolf, Mr. D. K. Yang.

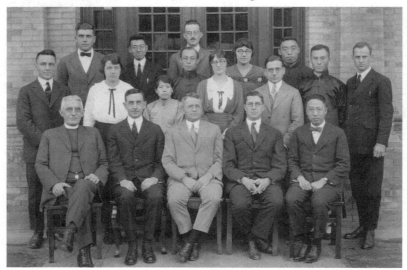

Ying Compound, Residence of PUMC Director

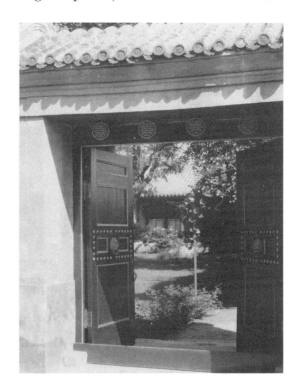

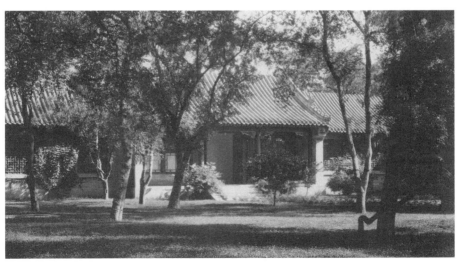

Prince Yu's Palace

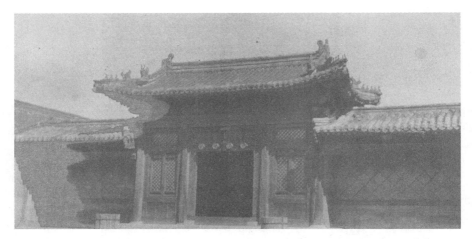

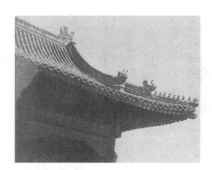

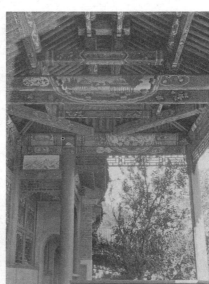

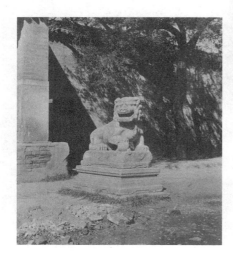

Peking Union Medical College

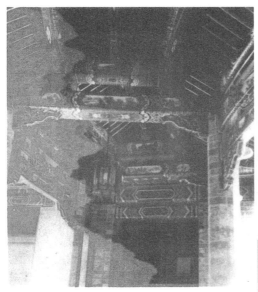

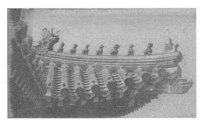

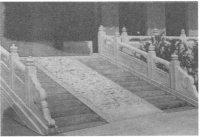

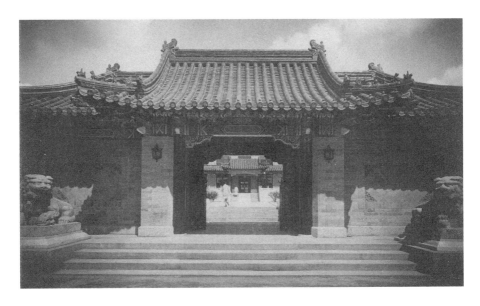

Faculty Residence Compounds

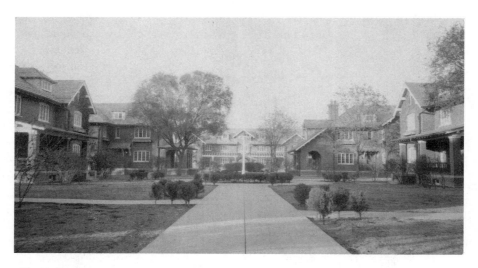

North Compound

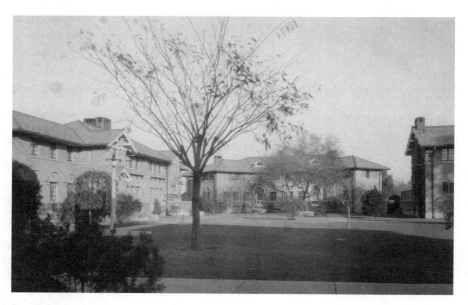

South Compound

Dedication—September 15-21, 1921

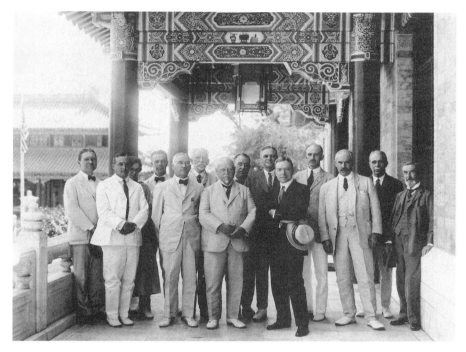

The Trustees: *Left to right*, Dr. Francis W. Peabody, Dr. Henry S. Houghton, Miss M. K. Eggleston, Mr. Edwin R. Embree, Dr. Paul Monroe, Dr. James L. Barton, Dr. William H. Welch, Dr. Richard M. Pearce, Dr. George E. Vincent, Mr. John D. Rockefeller, Jr., Mr. Roger S. Greene, Mr. F. H. Hawkins, Mr. Martin A. Ryerson, Dr. Christie Reid.

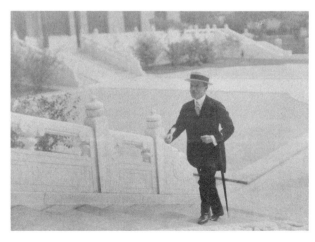

Mr. Rockefeller on steps of the Administration Building.

Dedication (*continued*)

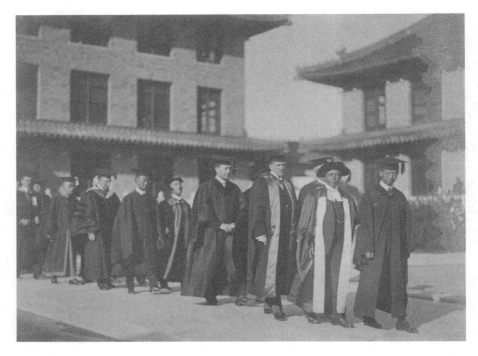

Right to left, Dr. W. S. New, Dr. Wu Lien-teh, Dr. K. Digby, Dr. J. E. Gossard, Dr. A. Sison.

President Hsü
Shih-ch'ang of
the Republic of
China greeting
Mr. Rockefeller.

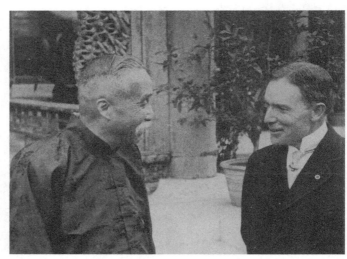

Dedication (*continued*)

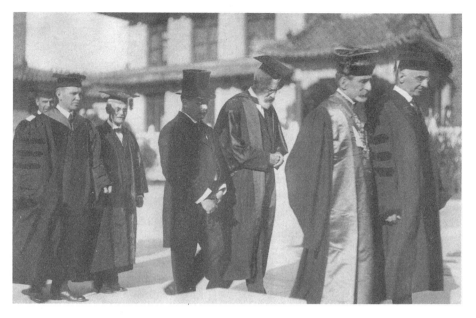

Left to right, Dr. Peabody; Sir William Smyly, *Dublin*; Dr. Thomas Cochrane, *London*; Dr. W. B. Macallum, *Montreal*; Dr. Tuffier, *Paris*; Dr. Victor G. Heiser.

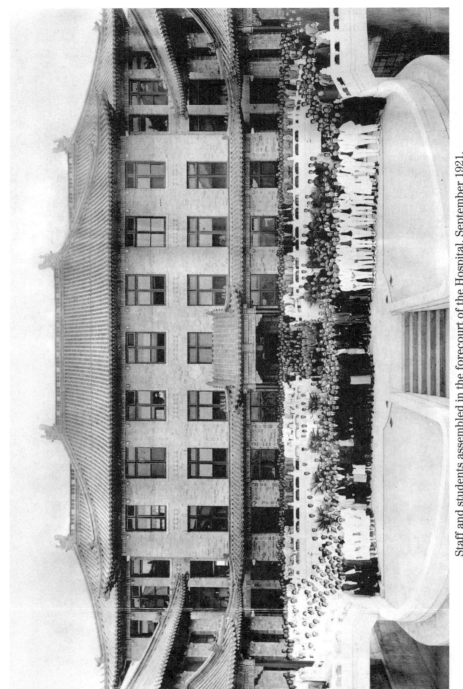

Staff and students assembled in the forecourt of the Hospital, September 1921.

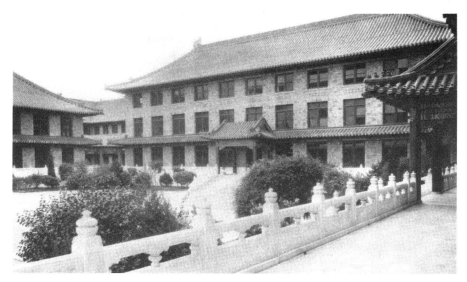

The Main Court of the Medical School

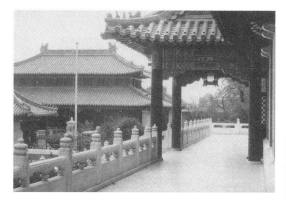

The Auditorium

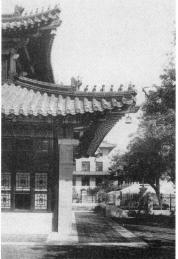

Roof Lines

Hospital Buildings

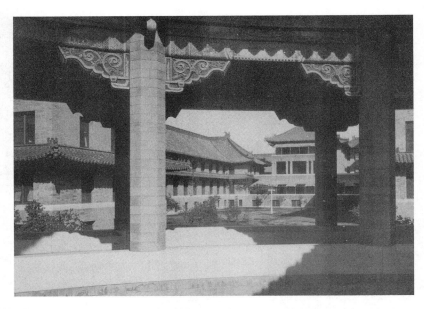

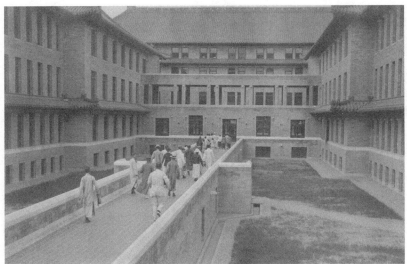

First Commencement—June 1924

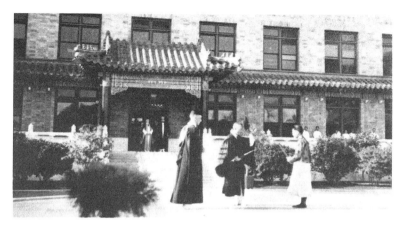

Establishing Tradition—Dr. Jerome P. Webster, *Chief Marshal*; Mr. Leslie R. Severinghaus, *Assistant Marshal*; Mr. Liu Shu-wan, *Student Marshal*.

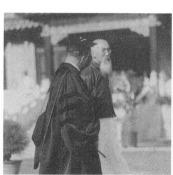

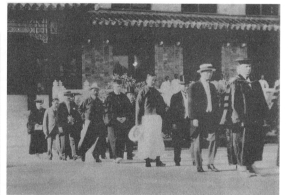

Dr. Houghton and Premier Sun Pao-ch'i.

Distinguished Guests.

At right, Tseng Hsien-tsang— first nursing graduate steps into place behind the Student Marshal. *Far right*, Liang Pao-p'ing, Liu Shao-kuang and Hou Hsiang-ch'uan, first medical graduates.

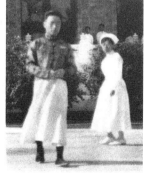

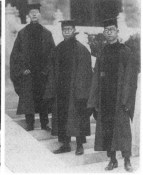

Funeral of Dr. Sun Yat Sen

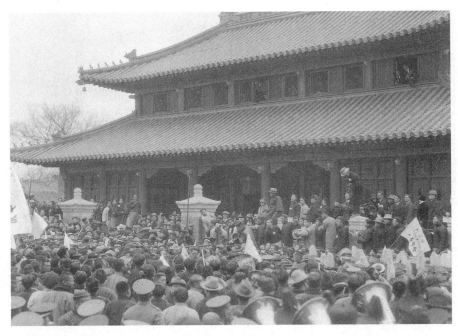

Crowds outside PUMC Auditorium where Christian services were held.

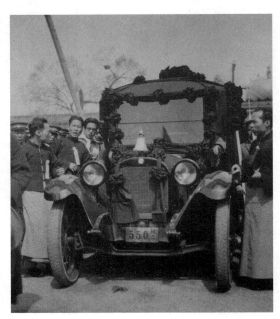

The PUMC truck, draped in black, which carried the coffin away from the Auditorium.

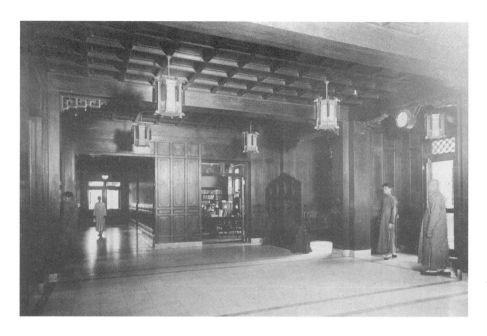

Lobby of Administration Building

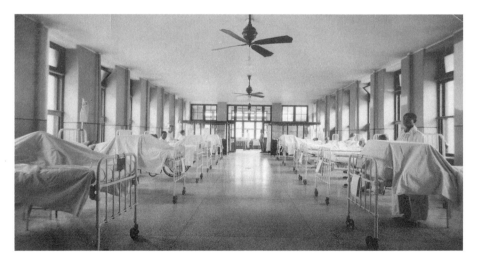

Typical hospital ward

Chairmen of PUMC Board of Trustees

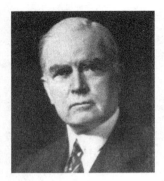

John R. Mott
1916-1920

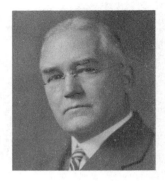

Paul Monroe
1920-1926—also Chairman
of CMB 1928-1934

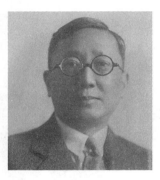

Sao-ke Alfred Sze
1926-1929, 1944-1946

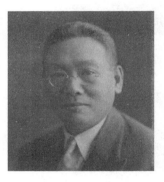

Y. T. Tsur
1929-1939

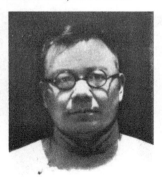

Sohtsu G. King
1939-1944

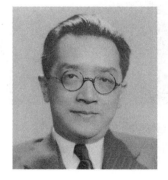

Hu Shih
1946-1949

CONTENTS

1

PREFACE I

"The work of the PUMC is among the bright jewels in our crown," wrote Raymond B. Fosdick, then-President of the Rockefeller Foundation, to Mr. Rockefeller, Jr. in 1945. The establishment of the China Medical Board (CMB) in 1914 marked the beginning of a transformative era in medical education and healthcare development across China. As we celebrate CMB's 110th anniversary, we are reminded of the profound impact it has had, particularly through its foundational and sustained support for the Peking Union Medical College (PUMC), which was modeled after the framework of the Johns Hopkins University School of Medicine. CMB takes great pride in how far PUMC has come, consistently upholding its high standards and continuing to serve as a beacon of excellence in medical education and healthcare.

It is within this context that CMB has undertaken the republication and retranslation of *China Medical Board and Peking Union Medical College*. Originally published in 1970, the English version of this work has long been out of print. By reintroducing this seminal text, we seek to revive its content and reaffirm the enduring story of CMB and PUMC as a model of U.S.-China collaboration in health and the humanities. The origins of this book are deeply rooted in the philanthropic vision of the Rockefeller Foundation, which foresaw the transformative potential of modern medicine.

The narrative within this book recounts the numerous challenges and triumphs encountered during the establishment and development of PUMC. It details the uncertainties of wartime, the complexities of administration involving multiple stakeholders, and the financial and political hurdles that had to be overcome. This historical journey exemplifies the tenacity and resilience needed to achieve such a monumental task, aptly described by Mr. Fosdick as "man against destiny, ideas that survived defeat"—a testament to the indomitable spirit that has driven human progress.

This book highlights how transformative advancements in medicine often require the courage and vision of individuals who face immense challenges. It underscores the contributions of early pioneers, administrators, and countless dedicated figures who played pivotal roles in the establishment and growth of PUMC. Their commitment was crucial in realizing PUMC's grand vision, demonstrating the profound impact determined individuals can have on medicine. Moreover, PUMC's faculty and graduates were pioneers in China, introducing key clinical specialties and innovative health systems, while also bringing their expertise to the global stage. Figures like Drs. Franklin C. McLean and Paul C. Hodges, who spent years working at PUMC, later became academic leaders at the University of Chicago, exemplifying the invaluable experience gained at PUMC and the global impact of these outstanding individuals, transcending national boundaries.

Looking back, we recognize the invaluable importance of firsthand experience. The Rockefeller Foundation and CMB's direct engagement with China was essential in truly understanding China's needs and challenges. Today, the promotion of people-to-people exchanges between the U.S. and China is more crucial than ever. Encouraging individuals, especially young people, to engage in cross-cultural and academic exchanges can foster mutual understanding and collaboration, building bridges for a better future. This book offers valuable historical insights to Americans, especially the younger generation, inspiring them to carry forward the spirit of their predecessors. Equipped with a solid education and an open mind, they can pursue personal growth and make meaningful contributions to society.

As we look to the future, CMB remains steadfast in its commitment to advancing health professional education, health policy, public health and research in China and beyond. The legacy of the past 110 years invigorates our mission, ensuring that the spirit of collaboration and excellence that defined our beginnings continues to guide us toward a healthier world. On the occasion of CMB's 110th anniversary, we hope that the republication of the English version and the revised Chinese translation of this book will enable a wider audience to explore the rich history of collaboration between PUMC and CMB, and to benefit from the insights and lessons it provides.

Wendy O'Neill
Chair of the China Medical Board Trustee Board

Roger I. Glass
President of China Medical Board

Barbara J. Stoll
Executive Vice President of China Medical Board

PREFACE II

"A history of Peking Union Medical College (PUMC) is half that of modern medicine in China." Over a century ago, PUMC was the first to introduce scientific medicine to the Chinese landscape, laying the humanitarian foundation through the name of science, and leading the glorious journey of modern medicine in China. Behind this remarkable history lies the visionary foresight of the Rockefeller family, whose efforts laid the cornerstone for PUMC's establishment. As an instrumentality of the Rockefeller Foundation, the China Medical Board (CMB) was initially tasked with establishing a medical college in China, comparable with the best medical schools in the U.S. and Europe, which was modeled after the framework of the Johns Hopkins University School of Medicine. Throughout this journey, despite encountering numerous difficulties and challenges, PUMC colleagues upheld the distinct Chinese spirit of resilience, remaining steadfast in their pursuit of the lofty ideals for medicine. With the guidance and support of the Chinese government, as well as assistance from the international communities, PUMC has forged an enduring legacy. Today, PUMC continues to play a pivotal role in collaborations in medicine and people-to-people exchanges, thanks to its rich historical heritage, outstanding medical expertise, and broad global vision. PUMC stands an epitome of goodwill between nations, a model of international and non-governmental assistance, and a vivid interpretation of international humanitarianism.

The deep and longstanding friendship between PUMC and CMB has set an exemplary model for the international collaboration between the U.S. and China in the field of health. Over the years, CMB has engaged in extensive collaboration with various Chinese institutions across multiple fields, including medical education, public health, nursing, and global health. On the occasion of the 110th anniversary of CMB, we are honored to be invited to write this foreword for the revised edition of *China Medical Board and Peking Union Medical College*. The author, Mary E. Ferguson, draws upon her firsthand experiences and unique perspective to transport us back to that tumultuous era. Ferguson, who worked at PUMC from the 1920s to the 1950s as the Secretary of the Trustees, has a deep understanding of the early years of PUMC. With meticulous detail, she chronicles the challenges of PUMC's founding, including the uncertainties of wartime and the clash of cultural ideologies. She also illustrates the extraordinary journey of PUMC, where, under the steadfast guidance of visionary leaders, resources were integrated, cutting-edge concepts and technologies were introduced, and generations of outstanding professionals with global vision, profound medical expertise, and exceptional leadership were nurtured. Additionally, Ferguson details the complex tripartite relationships among the Rockefeller Foundation, CMB, and PUMC, grounding her narrative in extensive archival research. These archives, considered among the richest sources of modern Chinese history in the U.S., make this book an essential read for anyone seeking to understand the intricate history of PUMC and CMB.

The 2014 Chinese translation made every effort to faithfully present the content of the original work. However, due to the limitations of the resources available at that time, there were still areas for improvement. With this in mind, and with the goal of further refining the translation in terms of faithfulness, expressiveness, and elegance, CMB and PUMC have worked closely together to lead a complementary translation team. This team has fully leveraged various resources, invited Chinese and U.S. history experts to provide insights, even traveling to the Rockefeller Archive Center in New York to verify historical facts. Additionally, the text has undergone further refinement to ensure that it is accustomed to local audiences while accurately reflecting the professionalism of the original work.

As the subtitle of this book—*A Chronicle of Fruitful Collaboration*— suggests, the partnership between PUMC and CMB attests to the importance of international exchange and collaboration. Today, China is thriving in the field of medicine, showcasing strong innovation. As the leading medical institution in China, PUMC carries a unique historical mission and social responsibility. It will continue to draw on international best practices in medical education and professional development, serving as a vital platform to promote medical and cultural exchange and collaboration between China and the U.S.—this is the book's profound relevance and timely significance.

"Science for Humanity"—this is the spirit of PUMC. From this perspective, this book is a masterpiece of PUMC's medical history research and heritage. PUMC has always emphasized the enhancement of character and aesthetics, striving to foster intellectuals with a high sense of social responsibility and humanistic spirit. During its collaboration with CMB, PUMC's efforts in medical history research and cultural preservation are a vivid embodiment of this philosophy. In recent years, PUMC has continuously enriched its historical and cultural treasury, achieving a blend of tradition and innovation: from the meticulous curation of PUMC's history exhibition, to the restoration and protection of its historic campus; from the manifestation of the PUMC spirit, to the creation of statues honoring its esteemed pioneers; from the resounding of PUMC's pipe organ, to the artistic paintings of the "PUMC Gallery"— the achievements are too numerous to count.

This revised edition is the result of the sincere collaboration between CMB and PUMC. Moreover, it represents a shared commitment by China and the U.S. to building a global community of health for all and a community with a shared future for mankind. Thus, this foreword is written.

WANG Chen
President of Chinese Academy of Medical Sciences
President of Peking Union Medical College

ZHANG Shuyang
President of Peking Union Medical College Hospital
Vice President of Chinese Academy of Medical Sciences
Vice President of Peking Union Medical College

FOREWORD

T HIS STORY of the China Medical Board and the Peking Union Medical College—concise, crisp and moving—brings back to me memories of glorious achievement in a gallant cause. What a pity it had to end as it did! And yet I cannot believe that it failed.

In creating the Peking Union Medical College we were far wiser than we realized. The concept of modern medicine which was introduced there set in motion influences in China that cannot be stopped. The conflict of ideologies—what Gibbon called "the exquisite rancor of theological hatred"—does not relate to medicine, for health is something that all men desire, and there is no limited supply for which nations must compete. Modern medicine is one of the ties that bind the human race together regardless of ideologies and boundary lines. It is one of the rallying points of unity and is thus a foundation stone in the ultimate structure of a united society.

This is exciting reading—man against destiny, ideas that survived defeat.

RAYMOND B. FOSDICK

INTRODUCTION

This CHRONOLOGICAL ACCOUNT of the genesis and development of the Peking Union Medical College during the thirty-seven years that it was supported by the China Medical Board and The Rockefeller Foundation sets the background for understanding the performance and accomplishments of this extraordinary institution which so profoundly influenced medical education and practice in China and throughout East Asia. The administrative aspect of the story has been of special interest to one who was intimately involved in it for more than twenty years. Evaluation of accomplishments will be a rewarding venture for some other chronicler.

To the China Medical Board of New York, Inc., and its officers: Dr. Joseph C. Hinsey, Chairman; Dr. Oliver R. McCoy, Director and now President; Dr. Patrick A. Ongley, the present Director; and Miss Agnes M. Pearce, Secretary; I am deeply grateful for the privilege of preparing this record. The encouragement and helpful interest they have maintained throughout, individually and severally, and their patience with the slowness of the pace at which it too often proceeded, have been indispensable factors in seeing it through to conclusion.

There has been easy access to a wealth of documentary material in spite of the fact that it has not been possible to review the important records in the files of the College in Peking. As the New York office of the PUMC the China Medical Board carried on a continuous correspondence with the administrative officers of the College, acting in many matters on its behalf, and keeping voluminous files which included minutes of the Board of Trustees and other administrative bodies in Peking. Preserved intact by the CMB, these records were the matrix in which most of the details of this story were embedded. The archives of The Rockefeller Foundation to which Mr. Raymond B. Fosdick kindly introduced me when I first embarked on this project, have provided valuable confirmation of events and dates especially for the early years when separation of the records of the inter-related RF, CMB, and PUMC had seemed of minor significance. To the successive officers of the Foundation who allowed me continued access to the archives, and to its helpful reference staff I am greatly indebted. Mrs. Roger S. Greene generously turned over to me private papers of her husband covering the years of his association with the CMB and PUMC. This invaluable material is now in the Houghton Library at Harvard University together with Mr. Greene's other personal papers.

One great boon has been the opportunity of talking directly with many who at one time or another served on the staff of the PUMC. Space does not permit listing everyone with whom I talked and corresponded and whose recollections enriched the developing picture—but to one and all go my warmest thanks for their "remembrance of things past" and for the pages from albums which helped to fill gaps in the photographic record.

Most significant of all in setting the record straight has been the participation of key figures in PUMC history: the late Dr. Franklin C. McLean, first Director; Dr. Henry S. Houghton, his successor who served again in the years before Pearl Harbor; Miss Anna D. Wolf, first Dean of the School of Nursing; and Miss Gertrude E. Hodgman, Dean from 1930 to 1940; Dr. Stanley D. Wilson, who was with the Premedical School from the beginning as head of the chemistry department and then as Dean; and Mr. Raymond B. Fosdick, President of The Rockefeller Foundation 1936-1948, who was involved in most of the crucial decisions affecting the College. Without the readiness of each of them to read drafts of the history as it developed, to illuminate events in which they had had a part, to fill in from personal knowledge gaps in the written record, and to encourage carrying the story to the end, it might well never have been completed.

As originally envisaged by the China Medical Board, this historical record was to have been prepared in collaboration with Dr. Harold H. Loucks, who had just retired from the Directorship of the CMB and who had been Professor of Surgery at the PUMC both before and after World War II. This would undoubtedly have resulted in a book with greater emphasis on the scientific and educational accomplishments of the institution. Extended periods of ill-health prevented Dr. Loucks from participating in the writing. Fortunately, however, it was possible as the present account took shape to keep in close consultation with him in person, by correspondence and by telephone. Every page of every draft had the benefit of his wisdom and balanced judgment.

I am beholden also to Mr. Chauncey Belknap, counsel for China Medical Board of N. Y., Inc. and The Rockefeller Foundation; Dr. L. Carrington Goodrich, Professor Emeritus of Chinese, Columbia University; and Dr. M. Searle Bates, Professor Emeritus of Missions, Union Theological Seminary, each of whom took the time to review the manuscript in its final stage greatly to its benefit.

My indebtedness and my gratitude to all these staunch friends of the PUMC are unbounded. To whatever extent this book has merit it is thanks to them. Where it falls short or is in error, the responsibility is mine and mine alone. For us all it has been a labor of love.

MARY E. FERGUSON

New York City
September 1, 1970

PROLOGUE

Cᴌᴇᴀʀʟʏ, whatever Western medical science may have to offer China, it will be of little avail to the Chinese people until it is taken over by them and becomes a part of the national life. So we must look forward to the day when most, if not all, of the positions on the Faculty... will be held by Chinese; when the Board of Trustees... will include leading Chinese, and when such current support as the institution may need beyond that derived from tuition fees and such endowment as may be set aside by its founders, will be derived from Chinese gifts and governmental subsidies, as is the case with medical institutions of similar rank in other countries of the world. Let us then go forward with one accord towards the attainment of this objective which will make permanent the establishment on Chinese soil of the best in scientific medicine that the world can offer.

JOHN D. ROCKEFELLER, JR.
speaking at the
Dedication Ceremonies of the
Peking Union Medical College
September 19, 1921

Chapter I

BEGINNINGS

1913-1916

Historically, China shares with the International Health Division in being one of the two oldest interests of The Rockefeller Foundation, and the Foundation has spent more money in this country than in any other country except the United States. So begins the chapter titled *The Johns Hopkins of China* in Raymond B. Fosdick's fascinating *Story of the Rockefeller Foundation*, published in 1951.

It was in the first decade of the twentieth century that John D. Rockefeller's vast fortune began to be applied toward major long-term objectives for the public good as envisioned by his farseeing adviser, Frederick T. Gates. In 1901 the Rockefeller Institute for Medical Research was established with Dr. William H. Welch as President. The next few years saw the burgeoning of the Institute under the effective direction of Dr. Simon Flexner, the formation of the General Education Board and the Rockefeller Sanitary Commission, the successful launching and continued massive support of the University of Chicago culminating in the "final gift" of $10,000,000 in 1910, and the early unsuccessful and often painful efforts to set up a Rockefeller Foundation.

All this was not enough, however, to satisfy the wide-ranging spirit of Mr. Gates. In 1909 he induced Mr. Rockefeller to finance an Oriental Education Commission, headed by President Ernest D. Burton of the University of Chicago, "for the investigation of educational, social and religious conditions in the Far East." The Commission visited the Near East, India, Japan and Korea, as well as China, which was its real goal. Mr. Gates believed that with an expenditure of approximately $10,000,000, "we might ourselves perhaps establish in China a University, teaching no religion, but hospitable to all faiths, a University in fact and not in name only, teaching all that is taught in Western universities, offering itself as a model for the Chinese government and raising up teachers for the new Chinese education." To his disappointment the report of the Commission convinced him that his plan of a great university in China was "a dream not then possible of realization."

His interest in China continued nevertheless. Two years later, in 1911, the success of the worldwide hookworm campaign, which carried with it the spread of scientific medicine and sanitation, seemed to point to a new and more promising direction. "Might we not do in medicine in China what we had failed in our attempt to do in University education? Might we not indeed at once attempt scientific medicine in China?"

For the moment such dreams had to be held in abeyance while all energies were bent to achieve the official incorporation of The Rockefeller Foundation. Once this was legally accomplished in May of 1913, the newly elected Trustees, all of whom had been actively concerned with the earlier events, lost no time coming to the conclusion that "the advancement of public health through medical research and education, including the demonstration of known methods of treating and preventing disease, afforded the surest prospect" of producing the "permanent and far-reaching usefulness" which was their aim. By the end of June, the International Health Commission of the Foundation had been set up to take over and expand the work which the Rockefeller Sanitary Commission had so effectively initiated in 1909.

What next? Public health, medical education and research were in the forefront of the Trustees' thinking. Two of the trustees—Frederick T. Gates and Jerome D. Greene —had a special interest in the Far East as a field for action; inquiries were coming from individuals interested in one or another project in China, and specific appeals had been made by the Executive Committee of the Harvard Medical School of China.[*] The time

---

[*] This young, struggling institution had the blessing of Harvard, but no organic connection or financial backing from the alma mater of the small group of altruistic Harvard graduates who had started it in 1911.

was ripe to seek an answer to Mr. Gates' earlier question — "Might we not... attempt scientific medicine in China?"

At a meeting on October 22, 1913, Mr. Greene, Secretary as well as member of the Board of Trustees, read a memorandum entitled *Educational and Other Needs in the Far East* in which he summarized a number of projects "having to do with education in the Far East, including medical education and the need of good hospitals," which had formally or informally been brought to the attention of the Foundation. He emphasized especially the application from the Harvard Medical School of China which had come through President Charles W. Eliot of Harvard University. Mr. Greene remarked that "a study of the whole question... would seem to be absolutely necessary if money is to be spent to the best advantage for medical work in China... The same statement holds good with regard to educational projects." The memorandum concluded with the comment that there seemed to be "subject matter sufficient to justify the most thorough consideration by a special commission to be sent to the Far East for this purpose."

The China Conference

Mr. Greene's suggestions were not immediately acted upon, but they were extensively discussed by the Trustees on December 20, 1913. This resulted in authorization for the Secretary "to call a conference on or about Monday, January 19, 1914, to consider medical and educational work in China and to invite to that conference, in addition to the members of The Rockefeller Foundation... such other persons as the officers should think it wise to invite." Invitations went from Mr. John D. Rockefeller, Jr. to the executive officers of the principal missionary boards, several medical missionaries, and other American residents of China who happened to be in the United States. Representatives of the Foundation and General Education Board also attended the conference which was held in the offices of The Rockefeller Foundation. The roster of those present is impressive: Mr. Frederick T. Gates, President Harry P. Judson, Dr. Simon Flexner, Mr. Starr G. Murphy, Dr. Wickliffe Rose, Mr. C. O. Heydt, Dr. Wallace Buttrick, Dr. Abraham Flexner, Mr. Jerome D. Greene, President Charles W. Eliot, Dr. Robert E. Speer, Dr. Henry W. Luce, Dr. Randolph T. Shields, Mr. James H. Franklin, Dr. W. H. Jefferys, Dr. John R. Mott, Dr. Charles D. Tenney, Professor Ernest W. Burton, Professor T. C.

Chamberlin and Professor C. R. Henderson, the three latter all from the University of Chicago, and Professor Paul Monroe of Columbia University. If such a conference were called today it would include a goodly number of Chinese participants; the fact that there were none is a striking example of how times have changed in the course of fifty years.

The exploratory nature of the meeting was set clearly by Mr. John D. Rockefeller, Jr., in his introductory remarks:

> The Rockefeller Foundation, which I presume is the host on this occasion, is a very small child, very young and inexperienced; it has the world as its field and it has very few plans; it is planning to go very slowly in laying out its work, and our thought has been to get all the information we can with reference to the different eligible fields, so that when we do arrive at some conclusion as to a point of attack, we feel that we know all that can be known about the problem involved, and that we are acting under the best advice obtainable ... We haven't any plans, we are not committing ourselves to anything in China or any place else... We simply state that there is a great opportunity, a great need. Now let us study the situation and see whether there devolves upon this Foundation a responsibility in this particular country.
>
> This office has been interested for some years in the problems of China—interested as a simple student—and we have felt that the great changes which were taking place in China were presenting opportunities which have never existed before and which, perhaps, the Foundation should consider.
>
> We are simply seeking information and I want to make it very clear at the outset that we have not determined to do something in China.

Mr. Greene presented an outline of topics under the two major headings, *Education* and *Medical Education and Public Health*, emphasizing that the immediate purpose of the conference was not "to determine action" but rather, through discussion to illuminate the question confronting The Rockefeller Foundation. "If a consensus of opinion should be developed as to a few clear-cut propositions, well and good; but the conference will have accomplished its purpose if it throws light on the general problem, whether by disclosing facts or even divided opinion as to facts or policies."

There followed two days of lively and fruitful talk. The stenographic record of the conference gives vivid evidence of the intense interest of this group of distinguished men in the challenge before them. Mr. Rockefeller was a skillful chairman, calling on one or another to open the discussion of each topic, and then giving opportunity for comments and expression of differing points of view. At the end of the second day, he brought the conference to a close with a warm expression of appreciation for the frank and constructive discussion which had provided so much information and so many ideas to The Rockefeller Foundation as it faced the formulation of its program.

The conference had been timed for the two days immediately preceding a meeting of The Rockefeller Foundation Trustees on January 21, 1914, to which those Trustees who had taken part in the discussions were able to bring firsthand impressions and comments. After due deliberation, the following decisions were reached by the Trustees:

1. that any work in China should be in medicine, and
2. that whatever might be undertaken should be based on existing agencies whether missionary or governmental.

At this meeting, President Eliot of Harvard, who had taken such an active part in the preparatory conference, was elected a Trustee of the Foundation.

A week later, January 29, 1914, Mr. Gates' reactions to the conference discussion were presented in the form of a paper entitled "The Gradual and Orderly Development of a Comprehensive and Efficient System of Medicine in China," a document which the Trustees adopted forthwith as the basis for immediate and future action. The plan outlined four steps:

STEP I   the mastery of existing data in the United States, England and Europe and the sending of a "carefully chosen and thoroughly qualified man to China at once to make and currently report a Survey of Current Medical Work and Education."

STEP II   on the basis of the data thus secured "to choose that medical district or province which seems best to lend itself to our purposes," the most important element being a large, well-equipped, well-conducted, and efficient medical school associated with a good hospital.

STEP III to ensure that there are adequate doctors and nurses and equipment in every hospital in the chosen area; to put the medical school simultaneously on the best practicable basis in men, equipment, hospital facilities and clinical material; to set up a program of visiting professors from abroad; to provide that every medical practitioner "on foreign pay" spend at least three months of every year at this central medical school—"this to be the unique, central and indispensable condition of work in China;" and to establish concurrently proper nurses' training schools for men and women.

STEP IV   to extend the system to other similar centers as it proves practicable and efficient.

Having adopted Mr. Gates' plan, the Trustees agreed at the same meeting to ask President Harry Pratt Judson of the University of Chicago and Dr. Francis W. Peabody of the Peter Bent Brigham Hospital in Boston to go to China and make the "Survey of Current Medical Work and Education" called for in Step I .

The First China Medical Commission

With the acceptance by Dr. Judson and Dr. Peabody of this challenging assignment, it seemed desirable to round out the Commission with someone, not necessarily a medical man or an educator, who had some familiarity with China. Several persons were mentioned, but there soon was general agreement on Roger S. Greene, then American Consul-General in Hankow, if he could get a leave of absence from the U.S. Department of State. Mr. Greene was warmly endorsed by Mr. Rockefeller, Jr., Mr. Gates, President Eliot, and President Judson. The only objection came from the Secretary of the Foundation, Jerome D. Greene, who dreaded mixing family relationships with business affairs and had previously resisted suggestions from Mr. Rockefeller that his brother might be a useful member of the working staff of The Rockefeller Foundation. In the end, the government leave of absence having been granted and his brother's objections withdrawn, Roger S. Greene accepted appointment as the third member of what came to be known as the First China Medical Commission. On April 19, 1914, he joined Dr. Judson, Dr. Peabody, and Mr. George B. McKibbin, Secretary to the Commission, in Peking. This was the beginning of twenty years in which he was to devote all his energy and ideas to the China Medical Board and the Peking Union Medical College. *

Armed with letters of introduction from the Chinese Chargé d'Affaires in Washington, which they promptly presented, the members of the Commission were cordially received by President Yuan Shih-k'ai and Vice President Li Yuan-hung, as well as other important officials.

Without delay they embarked on a study of the situation by visiting medical schools and hospitals in Peking and Tientsin, then set out for similar activity in other parts of the country. During the next four months they covered an amazing amount of ground—Tsinan, Hankow, Changsha, Kiukiang, Nanking, Soochow, Shanghai, Hongkong, Canton, Swatow,

---

* Hereafter frequently referred to as the CMB and the PUMC.

Amoy, Foochow, numerous side trips and even Manila and Formosa. All these places were visited by one or more of the members each of whom kept a detailed journal as he went along.

The commission members found an extremely fluid situation. Wherever they went they were drawn into meetings and conferences with local officials as well as American and British medical missionaries who welcomed their ideas and possible support in raising the quality of medical education in China, a subject of major current concern in the Chinese Medical Missionary Association.

It was August 17, 1914, when the group joined forces once again — this time in Kyoto, Japan, to compare notes, discuss observations, and develop recommendations for future action. Six weeks later they sailed for New York, Mr. Greene accompanying his colleagues, and on October 21, 1914, the resultant report *Medicine in China* was presented to the Trustees of The Rockefeller Foundation in New York.

The outbreak of World War I in early August 1914 must have injected many uncertainties into the Commission's deliberations, but these are not reflected in the final report and findings, or in the actions of the Foundation which followed. The comprehensiveness of the presentation shows clearly in the chapter headings:

CHAPTER I	Health Conditions in China	Dr. Judson
CHAPTER II	Chinese Native Medicine and Surgery	Dr. Judson
CHAPTER III	Western Medicine in China	
1.	Practitioners of Western Methods	Dr. Judson
2.	Chinese Government and Private Medical Schools	Mr. Greene
3.	Missionary Medical Schools	Dr. Judson
4.	Education of Women Physicians	Dr. Peabody
5.	Non-missionary Medical Schools under Foreign Control	Dr. Peabody
6.	Locations Considered for Medical Education	Mr. Greene
7.	Report on Hospitals in China	Dr. Peabody
CHAPTER IV	Standards of Medical Education under Missionary Auspices. Teaching in Chinese or in English.	Dr. Judson
CHAPTER V	Dissection and Autopsies	Dr. Peabody
CHAPTER VI	The Attitude of the Chinese Government toward Western Medicine	Dr. Judson

The whole report is absorbing reading to anyone interested in the China of that day, but it is Chapters IX and X which are of prime interest here, since these recommendations were responsible for the creation of the China Medical Board and establishment of the Peking Union Medical College.

In summary, the Commission recommended that the Foundation should undertake medical work in China on a large scale "with the understanding that it will involve a long time and that during that time the Foundation should be the most important factor in China in the development of medical instruction;" that teaching should be on the "highest practicable standard," with English as the principal language of instruction for some time to come. The Commission expressed the opinion that the time was "not yet ripe for the organization of a large work in relation to the public health," or for the establishment of "an independent institution for research in China" but recommended encouraging research in the medical schools aided.

They went on to recommend that "the first medical educational work organized should be in the city of Peking... in connection with the Union Medical College* if suitable arrangements can be made," failing which it would be desirable to undertake "an independent work" in Peking. They estimated that this would involve capital expenditures between $595,500 and $695,500, and an eventual annual subsidy between $154,217 and $203,447. A "second principal medical work" was recommended for Shanghai with the establishment of a new institution which would co-operate with existing medical schools in and near Shanghai and would serve to "unite the medical educational forces and the principal hospitals of the entire lower Yangtze Valley contributory to Shanghai."

---

* A joint enterprise of the London Missionary Society, the London Medical Missionary Association, the American Presbyterian Missionary Society, the Methodist Missionary Society, the American Board of Missions (Congregational), and the Society for the Propagation of the Gospel.

There followed a list of "minor" proposals which included grants in aid to the Canton Christian College and the medical plans of the Yale Mission at Changsha; the establishment of two model tuberculosis hospitals; fellowships to enable "selected Chinese graduates in medicine" to go abroad for further study; scholarships for promising medical students in the medical schools which were being aided; development of hospitals in areas "tributary to the medical schools... aided by the Foundation;" encouragement in the training of nurses; fellowships to enable medical personnel of hospitals to spend three months each year in one or another medical school; fellowships for medical missionaries in China to undertake advanced study in the United States or Europe; visiting professors to lecture in the medical schools aided by the Foundation and elsewhere; the formation of an "advisory committee of medical men" in the United States, and "if circumstances warrant, a similar committee in Great Britain"; and finally, "that the Foundation be represented in China by a Resident Commissioner, who will administer the affairs of the Foundation in connection with the institutions aided" with Peking as his headquarters.

The report was received with appreciation by the Trustees, who gave it the careful study that such far-reaching proposals demanded. At a meeting of the Foundation on November 5, 1914, called for the purpose of considering the report, the recommendations of the Commission were adopted as a working basis "subject to such changes and emendations as experience and further knowledge shall from time to time invite," and on November 30 it was voted "that an organization be created to take up medical work in China as recommended by the Commission and that such organization be designated the China Medical Board of the Rockefeller Foundation".

Establishment of the China Medical Board

No time was lost. On December 11, 1914, the China Medical Board of the Rockefeller Foundation met for the first time with Mr. John D. Rockefeller, Jr., in the chair. The charter members were a notable group of men:

DR. WALLACE BUTTRICK	MR. JEROME D. GREENE
DR. SIMON FLEXNER	DR. HARRY PRATT JUDSON
MR. FREDERICK T. GATES	MR. JOHN R. MOTT
PRES. FRANK T. GOODNOW	MR. STARR J. MURPHY

DR. FRANCIS W. PEABODY   MR. WICKLIFFE ROSE
MR. JOHN D. ROCKEFELLER, JR.   DR. WILLIAM H. WELCH

Mr. Rockefeller, Jr., was the Board's first Chairman; Dr. Buttrick its first Director.

They began at once to implement the recommendations of the Commission, starting with fellowships for Chinese medical graduates and for Chinese women to be trained in the United States as teachers of nursing and superintendents of nurses. The first purchase of land in Peking was also approved at this initial meeting of the Board—the beautiful old Chinese house which came to be the PUMC Director's residence and was known to all who were ever connected with the institution as the "Ying Compound." The meeting ended with the reading by Mr. Gates of a paper entitled "Thoughts on Medical Missions and the Spirit and Teaching of Jesus" and a discussion "as to the expediency of using this paper wholly or in part as an expression of the spirit and aims of the Board." No formal action to this effect was recorded, but the ideas expressed by Mr. Gates recur, sometimes almost word for word, in various later official statements.

From then on things moved quickly. Mr. Roger S. Greene was appointed Resident Director in China, and along with Dr. Buttrick began discussions in New York with the Secretaries of the American missionary boards cooperating with the London Missionary Society in the Union Medical College at Peking on the recommendations of the Commission affecting that institution. On March 15, 1915, a letter from Mr. Rockefeller, Jr., drawing heavily on Mr. Gates' paper, went to all missionary bodies in the United States then conducting medical work in China, outlining briefly the origin of the Board, and summarizing the steps "which the Foundation might find it desirable" to take in carrying out its comprehensive plans. These included assistance in strengthening existing medical schools and hospitals and their personnel, as well as "to establish, equip and support new medical schools and hospitals." Perhaps the most significant feature of this letter was Mr. Rockefeller's statement that in choosing personnel for independent schools or hospitals, the Foundation agreed "to select only persons of sound sense and high character, who were sympathetic with the missionary spirit and motive, who were thoroughly qualified for their work professionally, and who would dedicate themselves to medical ministration in China." Beyond these qualifications, however,

26

it could not "properly impose tests of a denominational or doctrinal nature, such as were deemed desirable by Missionary Boards for their own medical missionaries or agents." As the years went by, Mr. Rockefeller more and more looked back upon this letter as a personal commitment to the mission boards to maintain the Christian character of the institution— a conception which not only influenced future administrative policies but vitally affected the careers of some individuals.

Establishment of the Peking Union Medical College

Out of the numerous consultations of that period, in London as well as New York, came the historic agreement with the London Missionary Society whereby the China Medical Board purchased for the sum of US$200,000 the property of the Union Medical College in Peking, which was to be known thereafter as the Peking Union Medical College. On July 1, 1915, the China Medical Board assumed full support of that College which had an annual budget of $53,000. In due course representatives to serve on the thirteen-member Board of Trustees were appointed by the several mission boards and the China Medical Board. The PUMC board held its first meeting in New York on January 24, 1916, under the chairmanship of Dr. John R. Mott. From then on the Trustees assumed responsibility for the internal administration of the College. The China Medical Board handled the Trustees' requests for appropriations but dealt directly with its own Resident Director on land purchases and the building program of the College, and with his advice acted on other facets of the total program such as grants to other institutions and fellowships.

Under the agreements with the mission boards when The Rockefeller Foundation took over the Union Medical College, the China Medical Board was to appoint seven of the Trustees of the PUMC, the other six to be named by the individual mission boards. The seven representatives of the China Medical Board were all members of the CMB, and four of them also of The Rockefeller Foundation. For some time to come there was a very definite interlocking in the membership of these three boards. Small wonder if at times it became difficult to tell where final authority lay. In addition, the CMB and the PUMC Trustees functioned to begin with from Dr. Buttrick's office in the General Education Board where only an estimated 30 per cent of the staff's time was devoted to the work of the new boards.

The Second China Medical Commission

Dr. Buttrick was quick to recognize that the magnitude of the project on which the Board had embarked called for a measure of professional competence and experience which he, a Baptist minister, did not claim. He was convinced that if the agreed-upon program of medical education in China was to succeed, the situation should be studied on the field by the very best medical men possible. As far as he was concerned, this meant none other than his good friends and colleagues, Dr. William H. Welch and Dr. Simon Flexner, probably the two most important figures in American medicine at that time. Dr. Buttrick was both persistent and persuasive and when the China Medical Board's Second China Medical Commission sailed for China on August 7, 1915, he was accompanied by Dr. Welch and Dr. Flexner, together with Dr. Frederick L. Gates of the Rockefeller Institute (son of Mr. F. T. Gates) as Secretary.

The first commission had caught the vision of what might be. It fell to the second commission to give that vision form and substance.

As could be expected, Dr. Welch and Dr. Flexner set their sights high. "The aim should be to create as good a medical college as can be found anywhere in Europe or in America... with an excellent staff of teachers, well-equipped laboratories and a good teaching hospital and dispensary... a training school for both male and female nurses." But first there was a moral obligation to close out the old Union Medical College with the maximum consideration for all concerned. Finding the students "quite unfitted by their lack of preliminary training and ignorance of English to participate in the new order of things," the Commission in consultation with Mr. Greene worked out plans for the transfer, class by class, of the 128 students to other existing institutions where they could complete their medical education. Due provision to cover additional costs to the students themselves and to the schools receiving them was also recommended. The Commission felt that the kind of leadership required for the new school would have to be sought largely outside the ranks of the original faculty. Some might be reassigned to other mission posts in China, while others, after study abroad, might return to the new faculty which must be built up for the PUMC.

The Commission then turned to such specific problems as requirements for admission, language of instruction, content of the medical curriculum and length of the course. There was full agreement that the admission requirements for the PUMC and for the school projected in Shanghai should follow "as nearly as practicable those now adopted by the majority of the better schools in the United States." This might make it necessary at the outset for the medical schools to provide their own premedical courses, but they foresaw that "a great and much-needed service... would be rendered to the broader educational work of the college and the cause of higher medical education in China by aiding certain colleges to supply the required training in the fundamental sciences." While recognizing the importance of continued study of Chinese in the medical school, the earlier decision that English should be the language of instruction was confirmed, since they were "convinced that it is impossible to train students properly in modern medicine through the medium of this tongue [Chinese]."

Believing that "everything should be done to develop the spirit of scientific inquiry which is probably only latent and not really absent" the Commission recommended that "in the choice of teachers special emphasis should be laid upon their capacity as investigators or to stimulate investigation, as such men are generally the best teachers and exert a stimulating influence upon both students and their colleagues... It goes without saying that in accordance with the announced aims and obligations of the China Medical Board the men selected as teachers will be in sympathy with the missionary efforts."

Out of their own experience, they urged that no attempt be made to start with a completely organized school, but that the example of Johns Hopkins Medical School should be followed, developing year by year until there were students in each class of the five-year course (which included a year of internship). They also called attention to the impossibility of maintaining "this higher order of medical school" on the low scale of missionary salaries, and stressed the importance of adequate pension provisions and other fringe benefits.

It could not have been easy for these busy and important men to give four months to this mission, but the course they charted guided the Peking Union Medical College to outstanding achievements and an influence extending far beyond the walls of Peking.

On January 24, 1916, at the initial meeting of the Trustees of the PUMC in New York, Dr. Welch reported the findings and recommendations of the Commission, and a few days later these were presented to the China Medical Board. Great appreciation and interest were expressed, but neither board took any action. Obviously there was such confidence in the judgment of Dr. Welch, Dr. Flexner and Dr. Buttrick, that it was simply a matter of following through on their ideas and proposals.

Chapter II

EARLY DEVELOPMENT

1916-1921

W ITH THE DISSOLUTION of the faculty and staff of the old Union Medical College, appointment of the first administrative officers for the new institution was urgently needed. Dr. Buttrick, Dr. Flexner, Dr. Welch and two mission board secretaries, Dr. North and Dr. Brown, had been appointed by the PUMC Trustees as a standing committee on faculty. The criteria which they conscientiously applied to prospective appointees served to underline the goal of excellence at which the college was aiming.

Serious thought was given to finding the right man to head the college in Peking, and also someone for the school projected for Shanghai. Should he be a man with experience and established reputation in medical education? Or, might a younger man of demonstrated ability and promise prove more flexible and resourceful in this pioneer experiment in a foreign land? Initial approaches in the first category having been unsuccessful, the choice fell upon Franklin C. McLean, an assistant resident physician at the hospital of the Rockefeller Institute. On June 20, 1916, the Executive Committee of the PUMC Trustees, acting on the unanimous recommendation of the standing committee, appointed this twenty-eight-year old scientist, six years out of medical school, to be "Professor of Internal Medicine and head of the Peking Union Medical College" at the munificent salary of $2,400 a year plus necessary traveling expenses. On July 13, 1916, less than a month after his appointment, Dr. McLean sailed from Vancouver.

31

Accompanying Dr. McLean was Mr. Charles A. Coolidge, who had been appointed by the China Medical Board as "consulting architect." When the land and buildings of the old Union Medical College had been bought from the London Missionary Society, it was realized that these would be inadequate for the kind of institution the Board was hoping to develop. The Rockefeller Foundation had accordingly acted promptly when Mr. Greene cabled early in January 1916 recommending purchase for the sum of US$125,000 of the property of Prince Yu near the old Union Medical College. From then on the PUMC was commonly known as the Yu Wang Fu—Prince Yu's Palace. To many Chinese the name Rockefeller was synonymous with the Standard oil which filled their lamps, and since the word for oil sounds much like the name of the prince, it made an easy pun—the Oil Prince's Palace—a play on words which delighted the Chinese sense of humor.

Essential preparatory work for the new institution was an early architectural review of the properties now held by the Rockefeller Foundation in Peking. As with Dr. Welch and Dr. Flexner on the medical and scientific side, the China Medical Board chose its architectural consultant from the top rank in his profession. Mr. Coolidge was one of the leading American architects of that time, whose recent experience included planning and constructing the new buildings of the Harvard Medical School in Boston and of the Rockefeller Institute in New York. It was Dr. Simon Flexner who proposed his name and who prevailed on Mr. Coolidge to undertake this review.

Dr. McLean and Mr. Coolidge arrived in Peking on August 20, after a few days in Shanghai where Mr. Greene, Resident Director of the CMB and Dr. Houghton[*] had been their capable guides. On their way north they had also made brief stopovers at Nanking and Tsinan.

The following weeks were filled to overflowing with conferences, visits to numerous medical institutions, good and bad, missionary and government—always with the new Peking Union Medical College in mind.

---

[*] With the prospect of a Rockefeller Foundation supported medical school in Shanghai, the financially hard-pressed officers of the Harvard Medical School of China (see footnote on Page 14) had offered "to have its entire present work taken over at once and carried on" by the China Medical Board "until such time as the now proposed medical school is opened." The CMB had responded by buying the land owned by the Harvard Medical School of China; undertaking to complete the education "in the United States or elsewhere of recommendable students" then in the school; and most important of all, agreed to "engage the services of Dr. Henry S. Houghton," then Dean of the school.

Questions of who, if any, of the original staff of the Union Medical College might play a part in the future development of the new institution were still under consideration and Dr. McLean was immediately involved in weighing professional potentialities and qualities of temperament. With Mr. Greene he studied how best to handle the administration of the school in Peking in the light of its distance from the College Trustees in New York. Together they developed plans for the premedical department which both agreed must be established at an early date.

They decided to close forthwith the London Mission's Women's Hospital, poorly housed and equipped, as the Methodist Sleeper Davis Hospital for women, well housed and equipped, was available nearby.

The needs of the on-going Men's Hospital—X-ray facilities, laboratory service, pharmacy, business administration, nursing service—also required study. This hospital was staffed with male nurses, its training school open only to men. There was a widespread feeling in China that it was not possible to have women nurses caring for male patients. Most of the young women who served in hospitals for women had little preliminary education and minimal nursing training. Basically they served as aids to the "foreign" nurses, often being little more than servants given the most menial chores. At the Harvard Medical School of China in Shanghai, Dr. Houghton had pressed for the concept of nursing as an honorable profession to which young women of good education from families of standing in the community would be attracted, and could be assigned without question to the care of men as well as of women and children. A promising start had been made in the Harvard Medical School's teaching hospital, the Shanghai Red Cross Hospital. Wherever Dr. McLean and Mr. Greene went they discussed this question, receiving enough encouragement to confirm their own strong impression that one of the needs of first priority was the appointment of a Superintendent of Nurses to organize the nursing service of the new hospital and to prepare for training women nurses in a nursing school of the same high standard contemplated for the medical college.

Dr. McLean spent a full month in Peking, returning to Shanghai by way of the Yangtze Valley. In six weeks he had seen all the medical work of any significance in north and central China, and met most of the medical leaders—Chinese and Western. His final week, like his first, was spent in close contact with Mr. Greene and Dr. Houghton. Thus, at the very outset, these three young men—Dr. McLean, twenty-eight;

Mr. Greene, thirty-two; and Dr. Houghton, a venerable thirty-six—worked together laying the groundwork for the institution on which each of them was to leave his own significant imprint.

Architecture, Construction and Costs

Mr. Coolidge's stay in China was shorter than Dr. McLean's, but long enough to give a man of his experience an insight into the problems involved in constructing modern fireproof buildings suitable for the purposes of a first-class medical school and hospital. Dr. Flexner had pointed out to him before he left New York that all the buildings—hospital, dispensary, laboratories, dormitories and residences— "should bear relation to the country in which they are located, as well as to uses to which they are to be put;" that "expense of construction as well as expense of operation will prove serious considerations, both immediately and then ultimately when the costs of maintenance are faced;" and that "excessive and elaborate equipment in the laboratories and elsewhere would be unwise from the standpoint of upkeep and unwarranted from the point of view of original cost in a wholly philanthropic enterprise." No other specific terms of reference were given Mr. Coolidge although he undoubtedly knew that The Rockefeller Foundation on April 11, 1916, had authorized the sum of $1,000,000 for land, buildings and equipment for the Peking Union Medical College.

The beauty and strength in Chinese traditional architecture greatly impressed Mr. Coolidge. A few days after first seeing Prince Yu's Palace, he wrote "I have been sad ever since... at the thought that all those buildings with their carvings and color schemes should be destroyed." It was not surprising therefore that his preliminary report to the Board on returning to New York early in October included discussion of curved roofs of glazed tile from the standpoint of cost, practicability, and artistic appropriateness when combined with modern buildings more than one story in height. That he believed a satisfactory solution—apart from cost— could be worked out is evident from the sketches which accompanied this report, which show traditional Chinese tiled roofs.

Mr. Coolidge shared with Mr. Greene and Dr. McLean the hope that the Board would buy the so-called "Japanese property"* which separated

---

* On this property were a Japanese hospital, school and club.

the Yu Wang Fu and the Ying Compound. This would give an unbroken block of land stretching from Hatamen Street on the east to Shuai Fu Yuan on the west, and allow for future expansion. It was on this assumption that Mr. Coolidge planned his first layout, with the main entrance to the Medical School on Hatamen Street, and only the hospital buildings on the Yu property. From the standpoint of economy of administration and convenience in planning for the various services of the physical plant, he considered this "an ideal scheme and layout." It was with "great regret" that on his return to New York he learned that the Board felt enough money had already been spent on land and had decided against buying the additional property. His subsequent sketches were accordingly adapted to the more limited space of the Yu Wang Fu. (It is interesting to note that since the "nationalization" of the PUMC by the Peoples' Republic of China, this "Japanese property" has been added to the PUMC property, which now does cover the whole block as first contemplated by Mr. Coolidge).

While in China, Mr. Coolidge did not try to work out detailed cost estimates, but gathered all the information possible affecting costs. He recognized the bearing of wartime conditions—this was October 1916—on the availability and cost of such materials as must be imported. Freight prices had doubled; there was a great lack of ocean carriers; structural steel, plumbing fixtures, and other items would probably cost twice as much delivered as when bought in the United States. He was a realist, and even in his first report did not encourage the China Medical Board to believe that it would be possible to cover the land, buildings and equipment with the US$1,000,000 authorized by the Rockefeller Foundation.

When the Board met on December 22, 1916, they had Mr. Coolidge's figures, giving on a cubic foot basis his estimates of "what the buildings as shown on the sketch plan would have cost in America just before the war." These were reckoned on two hundred undergraduate students, excluding the fifth-year interns, and two hundred and sixty-eight hospital beds. Mr. Coolidge was not at the meeting, but in his covering letter he gave the opinion that "one-third more at least should be added to normal prices before the war to cover the present advance in prices." Without that added third, his estimated cost was US$3,214,068.

To a group of men who had been thinking in terms of one million dollars, this must have come as a great shock. The Minutes simply state that Mr. Coolidge's report was "discussed at length." In any case, they were receptive to considering what some other architect might say.

They did not have to look far for another opinion, nor wait long for it to be expressed. Mr. Harry H. Hussey, a partner in the architectural firm of Shattuck & Hussey with offices in Chicago and Peking, was actually in an anteroom while this discussion was going on, hoping he might be called in for comment. Mr. Greene and Dr. McLean had talked in Peking with Mr. Coolidge about the possibility, and in their opinion the desirability, of using Mr. Hussey to some extent in the planning and construction. They felt that it would be advantageous to have an architect on the spot with whom they could be in current consultation throughout the building process. They were impressed by Mr. Hussey's familiarity with local building conditions and problems, and by his enthusiasm for the whole project. A ware of all this, Mr. Coolidge's report touched on some of the administrative problems in a division of responsibilities between designing architects in the United States and supervising architects in Peking, but recognized that it was up to the Board to decide what it wanted to do. In the meantime, Mr. Hussey had come from Peking to press his interest.

According to the Minutes, Mr. Hussey was "invited to come into the meeting for conference... was introduced and, after conference, retired." The substance of the discussion is not recorded but from other material in the archives, Mr. Hussey evidently gave an estimate that if he were architect on the spot he could build these buildings for US$1,000,000. This obviously impressed the Board, for after Mr. Hussey left the meeting, action was taken appropriating $1,000 "for a study of and plans for two buildings at Peking, one for a hospital and one for a laboratory, to be presented by the architectural firm of Shattuck & Hussey," before the next meeting of the China Medical Board in January 1917.

On January 23, 1917, Mr. Hussey submitted a series of attractive sketches with layouts closely following those drawn by Mr. Coolidge. These were much more comprehensive than the two buildings asked for at the December meeting, and included his "rendition" of the completed plant with graceful tiled roofs and spacious courtyards, making an impressive show. Before the meeting ended, three important actions were taken: (1) approval of Messrs. Shattuck & Hussey "as the architects for the Peking Medical School;" (2) appointment of a Building Committee consisting of Dr. Buttrick, Dr. George E. Vincent, and Mr. Starr J. Murphy "for the construction of the proposed buildings in Peking at a cost of not to exceed one million dollars;" (3) a request to the Rockefeller Foundation to increase the original allocation of $1,000,000 by $365,000, to cover the amount already expended for purchase of land in Peking.

The fact that the United States was on the verge of entering World War I does not seem to have raised any serious doubts as to the feasibility of carrying through so ambitious a construction program any more than the outbreak of that war had deterred the First China Medical Commission from the far-reaching recommendations drawn up in mid-August 1914.

Dr. Winford H. Smith, Superintendent of Johns Hopkins Hospital, who had offered space in the new Children's Hospital at Johns Hopkins for Mr. Hussey and his draftsmen, was named consultant on the construction, and worked closely with Mr. Hussey and Dr. McLean. Mr. Coolidge was consulted from time to time but the responsibility for developing the plans was Mr. Hussey's.

From then on, however, there was a steady rise in cost estimates and actual expenditures. Increased costs of materials and an unfavorable exchange rate were contributing factors. By June 1917 the cost over and above the $1,365,000 already authorized was estimated at $250,000; in July the estimate was placed anywhere up to $500,000; by December the Building Committee recommended suspending construction on five units for the time being while a careful study could be made as to the future course of action. On finding that the proposed suspension would increase final costs still further, the Board decided that the total building program should be carried through to completion without interruption.

The unhappy situation was compounded by a growing realization in the CMB that the original contracts which had made one man both architect and builder, had been unwise. In May 1918, on recommendation of the Comptroller of The Rockefeller Foundation, following a visit to Peking, the two original contracts were cancelled. A new contract was made with Mr. Hussey as architect only, and the Board set up its own construction department in Peking.

Even so, costs continued to skyrocket. In December 1918 the total figure including land, buildings and fixed equipment, movable equipment, accessories, and the first books for the library came to the staggering total of $5,956,208. But the end was not yet. By February 1919 plans for the Shanghai school were indefinitely postponed which meant that Mr. Hussey's services as architect were no longer needed for that project, and his contract was duly terminated in accordance with its provisions for such termination. Still the need for additional appropriations continued. By December 1919 the total estimated cost had risen to $6,885,650. There must have been extended discussion and much heart-burning. At any rate, having put its hand to the plow, the China Medical Board had no choice but to go forward and The Rockefeller Foundation to meet its requests for further funds.

The final figure carried on the books of The Rockefeller Foundation for the cost of land, buildings and equipment of the PUMC was $7,552,836. At the time of the dedication of the College in September 1921, Mr. Vincent, in a newspaper interview, gave the following explanation of why the cost had been so high:

> Exchange alone cost us $1,750,000. Most of our purchases were made during the war and at war prices. Ocean freights were never higher. Some of our material was reported lost en route to China and we duplicated the order. Sometimes this was done only to have both shipments ultimately appear. The Board of Trustees had only two alternatives, either to close down on the building and allow the large staff already on the field to remain idle and disintegrate pending an uncertain time of peace, or to go ahead with the building in spite of the unusual difficulties. We had to make our choice.

And so, the million dollar plant proved to be a seven-and-a-half million dollar enterprise, making it necessary for The Rockefeller Foundation to give up its original plan for a second school in Shanghai.

The Shanghai Medical School of The Rockefeller Foundation

While the major part of the time and attention of the China Medical Board was devoted in the first years to the establishment and construction of the PUMC and to the strengthening of mission hospitals over a wide area of China, it was not forgotten that there was also a commitment to "a second principal medical work" to be established in Shanghai. A provisional charter from the Regents of the University of the State of New York was granted on April 12, 1917, to the Shanghai Medical School of The Rockefeller Foundation, followed by the organization of a Board of Trustees with eleven members, Mr. George E. Vincent, Chairman; and Dr. Buttrick, Secretary. One of this Board's first actions was to elect Dr. Henry S. Houghton Acting Dean of the Shanghai Medical School of The Rockefeller Foundation.

The China Medical Board made an initial appropriation of $25,000 for buildings and fixed equipment. The contract with Shattuck & Hussey for the planning and construction of the PUMC included the eventual development of plans for the Shanghai Medical School. Appropriations were made for an administrative budget, a beginning in the purchase of books for the library, further acquisitions of land, fixed equipment and accessories. Plainly, the China Medical Board was moving ahead with plans for the Shanghai school as fast as this could be done without impeding progress in Peking.

In the meantime, since Dr. Houghton had practically no current administrative responsibilities for the Shanghai Medical School, he was available to serve the China Medical Board in other ways. When Dr. McLean returned to the United States for war service, Dr. Houghton went to Peking to carry on in his place in the expectation of returning to Shanghai in due course. As Acting Director of the PUMC, he was deeply involved along with Mr. Greene in all the problems of the building program, so that he was well aware that the rising costs were likely to affect the amount available for the Shanghai school. Early in December 1919 he joined with Mr. Greene and Dr. Buttrick, at the request of the China Medical Board, in making "a special study of the possibility of maintaining in Shanghai a medical school of satisfactory grade upon a basis of minimum expenditure... and gradual development from comparatively small beginnings."

The results of that study were presented at a special meeting of the CMB on April 28, 1920. After a résumé of the various official acts and statements, several possible courses of action were suggested: (1) immediate construction; (2) indefinite postponement; and (3) complete abandonment of the project. Arguments in favor of continuing with the plans for the Shanghai school were carefully considered. The Minutes do not record the points—pro and con—but state simply that "after extended discussion" it was:

RESOLVED that it is the sense of this Board that the plans for a medical school in Shanghai should be abandoned and that the officers be requested to formulate for presentation at the regular May Board meeting resolutions to carry out this decision.

This must have been an agonizing conclusion to reach. Could The Rockefeller Foundation afford to abandon a project which had aroused such justifiable expectations, and resulted in plans and alterations of plans by other individuals or institutions? Granted there was no *legal* obligation to build a school at Shanghai, did a *moral* obligation exist?

It was agreed that final action must be taken by The Rockefeller Foundation of which the China Medical Board was only a specialized agency. On May 26, 1920, The Rockefeller Foundation adopted a statement announcing that "owing to changes in the world situation growing out of the war, it has felt impelled to set aside the purpose previously announced of establishing a medical school in Shanghai." Eight months later, on February 16, 1921, the Trustees of the Shanghai Medical School of The Rockefeller Foundation assembled for their fifth and final Annual Meeting, and took action dissolving the Board, surrendering its provisional charter and corporate rights.

As one reviews the pertinent records of that time—minutes, memoranda, correspondence, and the pages of the Chinese Medical Journal—one cannot escape the conclusion that the decision to abandon the plans for the Shanghai Medical College was inevitable, unhappy though it made many people, including Dr. Vincent and Mr. Greene. There were strong protests from President Eliot and others originally interested in the Harvard Medical School of China, who had looked forward to a new successor school in Shanghai. Some missionary leaders who had welcomed the prospects of the Shanghai school as relieving them of the need to undertake such a development themselves felt that they had not been fairly treated and were openly resentful.

Disappointing as the abandonment of the Shanghai project was, its effects were not all negative. For the medical school of St. John's University, this decision opened up a promising future. As the only medical school in Shanghai teaching in English, its goal of academic excellence was demonstrated over the succeeding years by the professional competence of its graduates which won the esteem of Chinese and Westerners alike. A cordial spirit of cooperation grew up between the PUMC and the St. John's Medical School, many of whose alumni went to Peking for specialized graduate training. The medical school also benefited indirectly from the China Medical Board's contributions to the science departments of the University which between 1917 and 1928 totaled US$98,000.

Another unanticipated positive result was described by Mr. Greene some years later as "the rounding out of the original plan for the development of modern medicine in China... in the development at last of a Chinese governmental institution, sympathetic with our aims and methods, and possessing the potentiality of a far-reaching influence through which larger results can be obtained from previous investments of the Foundation in China." He was referring to the National Medical College of Shanghai, a part of the Shanghai Medical Center, to which The Rockefeller Foundation in 1934 transferred the land purchased in 1920 for its abortive "second principal medical work." For nearly fifteen years this had been carried on the Foundation books at US$298,331.95. Its actual value increased so greatly that the proceeds from its eventual sale paid for a more convenient site at Feng Ling Chiao on the western fringes of Shanghai, construction of fine well-equipped buildings, with a substantial sum left over toward an endowment to supplement other sources of income. The National Medical College of Shanghai soon became one of the best of the Chinese medical schools.

The PUMC itself reaped one incalculable benefit—the group of men designated for the faculty of the Shanghai school, some of whom were temporarily on the staff in Peking while others were on fellowships in the United States, could now be held on the Peking faculty. It is to the Shanghai Medical School of The Rockefeller Foundation in which they never served, that the PUMC owed the years of productive service of such men as Henry S. Houghton, A. M. Dunlap, Adrian S. Taylor, Paul C. Hodges, Andrew H. Woods, and Harvey J. Howard.

The Premedical School

Arrangements for the premedical science teaching which Dr. Welch and Dr. Flexner had foreseen would have to be the responsibility of the medical school at the outset, were high on the list of priorities drawn up in the autumn of 1916 by Dr. McLean and Mr. Greene. While Dr. McLean was in the United States looking for suitable teachers in the basic sciences, Mr. Greene and the continuing faculty of the Union Medical College concerned themselves with finding students who might qualify for admission to what was then spoken of as the Preparatory Department. (The name Premedical School appears for the first time in the Minutes of the Annual Meeting of the PUMC Trustees on April 11, 1917, in connection with the appointment of the first group of instructors—no formal action on the name appears anywhere in the record).

Bulletins went out to all the leading colleges in China and many middle schools announcing that the preparatory department would open on September 11, 1917, and the medical school in the autumn of 1919. These included the significant statement that while "the College is not prepared at this time to admit women to its classes... it is the purpose of the Board of Trustees in due time to admit qualified women students to the medical school on the same basis as men." The first women were admitted to the Premedical School in September 1919 and to the Medical School in 1921. The PUMC was the first co-educational medical school in China.

Dr. McLean's sound judgment and his enthusiasm for the project brought together a fine group of teachers. The first two arrived in Peking in early September, Dr. W. W. Stifler, head of the physics department and first Dean of the Premedical School, and Dr. Stanley D. Wilson, head of chemistry. The laboratories and classrooms in Lockhart Hall (the main building of the old Union Medical College) had been readied for use, and on September 11, 1917, the Premedical School opened with eight students. Local appointees that first year were Mr. C. T. Feng in Chemistry, Mr. Y. T. Tong in Physics, Mr. L. Carrington Goodrich, English, and Mr. Ma Kiam, Chinese.

To the Premedical School faculty in the next few years came a number of able young men and women from the United States who later made their mark elsewhere in China and the United States. The complete roster appears in Appendix B.

It is of more than casual interest that when the search was being made for a Chinese "with a good classical education in his own language, who also possesses the modern point of view," Mr. Greene passed on to Dr. McLean a suggestion that a certain "Mr. Su Huh," working for a Ph.D. in philosophy at Columbia University, might be suitable. The files do not show whether "Mr. Su" was ever approached, but many years later, as Dr. Hu Shih (the romanization of his name which he had subsequently adopted), eminent philosopher, educator and diplomat, he served the College with distinction as Chairman of its Board of Trustees in Peking.

As the faculty expanded, so did the requests for admission, a situation which made it possible to be increasingly selective in the students admitted. In 1919, for example, some 64 candidates were examined in such widely-scattered cities as Peking, Shanghai, Wuchang and Taiyuanfu, of whom 26 were accepted. In 1923, 172 applications were received. Out of 136 presenting themselves for examination, 28 were admitted.

Concurrently, the China Medical Board embarked on a program of helping in the development of science departments in existing colleges and universities so that they could eventually provide adequate preparation for the study of medicine. These included St. John's University, Fukien Christian University, Canton Christian College, Ginling College, Yale-in-China, Peking (Yenching) University, the University of Nanking, Soochow University (all mission-supported); two Chinese government institutions, Southeastern University and Tsinghua College, and one private Chinese university, Nankai. The assistance was varied—buildings, equipment, salaries for increased personnel; financing of an educational conference in Shanghai of interested mission boards; graduate fellowships for teachers in the natural sciences.

By the summer of 1925 the situation had so changed that the Premedical School could be closed. It had fulfilled its primary function of preparing the first students to enter the "first-class" Medical College which the Second China Medical Commission envisioned. Out of 205 individuals admitted, 100 went on to the Medical College and 84 completed the full five-year course leading to the coveted M. D. degree.

Of even greater importance was the demonstration which the Premedical School provided in the eight years of its existence in the teaching of the fundamental sciences at a high academic level, with emphasis on student participation in the laboratories. Soon, colleges and universities all over China were raising their own standards of science teaching, which inevitably affected standards in other fields. Thus, what started as an expedient for securing qualified students for the PUMC, actually had a far wider impact on higher education throughout China, and indirectly elsewhere in Asia.

Laying the Cornerstone

On September 24, 1917, just thirteen days after the first eight students entered the Premedical School, the cornerstone of the new Peking Union Medical College was laid in the southern foundation wall of what was to be the Anatomy Building. Dr. Paul S. Reinsch, American Minister to the Republic of China, presided; the speakers were Dr. McLean, "head" of the new institution; Dr. Frank S. Billings, Dean of Rush Medical College in Chicago where Dr. McLean had studied medicine, currently a Lt. Colonel of the U.S. Army Medical Corps in charge of the American Red Cross Mission to Russia; and Mr. Fan Yuan-lien, Minister of Education, who formally laid the stone. The Anglican Bishop of North China, the Rt. Rev. F. L. Norris, pronounced the benediction.

Dr. McLean reiterated the purpose of the Trustees "to establish here an institution devoted to medical teaching and research and the care of the sick, complete in every respect, and with the high standards of work that are already existent in the best of similar institutions abroad... Given the opportunity for study and research, this country should develop a medical profession to be proud of, and one that may easily take its place among the leaders of the world... It is the best of our modern medicine that we desire to give to China, that China may take advantage of our own recent progress."

The photographs taken that day give the real feeling of the occasion. The platform in the open courtyard for the speakers and other dignitaries, built around the base onto which the great square marble stone was lowered by a crane proudly operated by one of the Chinese construction men; the Marine band of the American Legation Guard playing from the terrace in front of the main palace building; the assembled guests, Chinese and Western, sitting in the warm autumn sunshine with the high tile-topped palace wall in the background and the participants standing on the steps of the Ancestral Hall of Prince Yu for the inevitable formal photograph; behind them the five-colored flag of the Chinese Republic. For a brief moment past and future met.

Building an Administration

Shortly after the laying of the cornerstone, Dr. McLean returned to the United States, taking with him an encouraging report on the state of the developing institution, recommendations for an interim administrative organization, and a draft worked out in Peking for the first Annual Announcement. The China Medical Board and the PUMC Trustees accepted these recommendations with satisfaction at the progress being made. In due course the Annual Announcement for 1918-1919 was published, its format and text following closely the draft brought from Peking except for some shortening of the introductory section covering the history and organization. How well the drafters had done their work is evidenced by the fact that this text and format was the pattern right up to 1941, subject only to the inevitable changes in a growing institution.

Dr. McLean now raised the question of his volunteering in the U.S. Army Medical Corps, telling Dr. Buttrick that he felt conditions in Peking justified his doing so. The building program was well underway, the Premedical School a going concern with a competent faculty, the old Hospital and Out-patient Department satisfactorily reorganized for service until the new buildings would be ready, and Mr. Greene and Dr. Houghton both thoroughly familiar with his own ideas as well as the thinking in New York. With some reluctance but with sympathy, the boards agreed to his request, and by the end of December he was at the Base Hospital in Camp Bowie, Fort Worth, Texas, in the uniform of a first lieutenant. It had been agreed that he would give such attention to PUMC affairs as was possible, and for the next six months there was a regular exchange of correspondence between Dr. McLean, the officers in Peking, and the New York office, with many decisions as to personnel and other matters being taken by him. Dr. McLean went to France in mid-July of 1918; from then until his discharge six months later with the rank of major, he was Director more in name than in fact, although still in touch with developments in both New York and China, and consulted on faculty appointments.

In the meantime the Trustees had responded to Mr. Greene's insistence that "Professor of Medicine and Physician-in-Chief" was hardly an accurate description of Dr. McLean's executive responsibilities, and had changed the title to "Director of the Peking Union Medical College."

As soon as it was clear that Dr. McLean would not be returning to Peking until the war was over, the PUMC Trustees, in response to Mr. Greene's cabled urgings, appointed Dr. Houghton Acting Director, a title which he carried until January 1, 1921 when he succeeded to the substantive post of Director from which Dr. McLean had resigned to devote his full time to the professorship of medicine.

The intervening three years had been filled with the problems and growing pains of any new institution, problems compounded a hundredfold by the miles that lay between New York and Peking. It took two months to get an answer to letters, and then only if they were dealt with promptly; the condensed language of cables often led to misunderstandings; administrative lines of responsibility were easily tangled between the three home boards, with their interlocking members and officers, not to mention a Director of the Medical College absent on military service but actively concerned in its affairs, an Acting Director in Peking, and a Resident Director of the China Medical Board whose responsibilities required him not only to travel in China but to return at intervals to the United States.

Years of problems—yes; but even more, years of progress and accomplishment. Notwithstanding the difficulties in the construction program, old buildings were renovated, new buildings took shape, faculty housing was pushed ahead for the growing numbers on the staff. The Pre-Medical School set up a curriculum and standards of achievement requisite for admission to the projected Grade A Medical College and sought students who could meet the challenge. On October 1, 1919, the Medical College admitted its first class of seven students, five of whom were graduates of the Premedical School. A year later the Nurses Training School was opened with three students; Miss Anna D. Wolf was its capable head. Pending the completion of the new hospital buildings the refurbished Men's Hospital of the old Union Medical College, its facilities expanded with the appointment of additional professional staff, continued to run to capacity, and to provide the clinical instruction for the last two classes of the former Union Medical College.

With so much going on, the importance of orderly administration increased. A Local Executive Committee had been set up by the Trustees in May 1916, supplemented a few months later by a committee to manage the Premedical School. As time went on and the faculty increased in numbers there were many hours of discussion, much of it informal and off-the-record, which showed a wide range of opinion on administrative organization. The first committee was replaced by an Administrative Board of which administrative officers and heads of academic departments were members. Standing Committees of the Administrative Board were set up to deal with Budget; Library; Fellowships and Scholarships; Admissions, Graduation and Curriculum; Bulletins and Announcements; Hospital; Graduate Study; Housing; and Women Students. The variety and range of these committees suggest that the final step had not yet been taken to distinguish clearly between matters of academic and professional concern and problems of fiscal and business management, although there was much wider participation in the developing program than before.

In the course of the next year Dr. McLean, now released from the army, engaged in scientific research at Harvard while simultaneously giving time and attention to PUMC matters such as appointments and problems of academic and administrative policy. It became increasingly clear to him as well as to his colleagues in Peking that the developing institution required a full-time Director. Should he, himself, continue in that post he would have to give up his teaching and research, something he was not prepared to do. On April 6, 1920, he submitted to the Trustees his resignation as Director in order to devote himself to the professorship of medicine.

Earlier that same week Dr. McLean had participated in one of the out-of-town conferences at Gedney Farms, New York, where the leaders of The Rockefeller Foundation and its related boards periodically gathered to thrash out problems and situations before they came up for formal Trustee consideration. Attending this particular conference were Mr. Vincent, Dr. Simon Flexner, Mr. F. T. Gates, Dr. F. L. Gates, Dr. H. P. Judson, Mr. Greene, Dr. Richard M. Pearce, Dr. Welch, and Mr. Edwin R. Embree, Secretary of both the China Medical Board and the PUMC Trustees. The discussion had centered chiefly around the basic purposes of the institution, the relative importance of teaching and research and their bearing on faculty appointments and advancement, the difficulty of defining policies and scope before budget limits had been set, all subjects about which considerable diversity of opinion had developed in both Peking and New York, and on which Dr. McLean himself had very strong ideas.

Dr. McLean had begun to fear that financial considerations were bringing the China Medical Board to a readiness to settle for a school of mediocre academic standards with emphasis on quantity rather than quality, and with too little emphasis on research. He made it very clear that such an institution held no attractions for him.

There was unfortunately no stenographic record of the discussion. Considering the participants, it must surely have been frank and forthright. It undoubtedly did much to clarify the thinking of the Board. Its most significant result was the formulation of the following statement, for the drafting of which Dr. McLean was primarily responsible, summarizing the scientific policy of the College, which received unanimous approval from the conferees:

Within the limits of the resources made available, the scientific aims of the Peking Union Medical College are:

1. Primarily to give a medical education comparable with that provided by the best medical schools of the United States and Europe, through
   a. an undergraduate medical curriculum;
   b. graduate training for laboratory workers, teachers, and clinical specialists; and
   c. short courses for physicians
2. To afford opportunities for research, especially with reference to problems peculiar to the Far East.
3. Incidentally to extend a popular knowledge of modern medicine and public health.

This statement, approved by the Trustees of the College on April 14, 1920, was never modified or changed in succeeding years, and continued to be a concise and accurate summary of the institution's scientific aims, as first expressed by Dr. Simon Flexner and Dr. William Welch, who also took part in this reaffirmation.

Conscious of the fact that the faculty in Peking felt they should have some say in the choice of Dr. McLean's successor, the Trustees left it to the Executive Committee "in consultation with the Administrative Board in Peking" to make recommendations to the Trustees "as to the Director to be appointed," and pending such recommendations simply continued Dr. Houghton as Acting Director. Of all Dr. Houghton's varied contributions to the College, perhaps the most important was his cheerful readiness in that first crucial period to carry whatever administrative responsibilities were asked of him, no matter how anomalous and indefinite his own situation might be. It is hard to see how without him the institution could have come through the difficulties, uncertainties, and crises which marked its beginnings.

One of the participants at the Gedney Farms Conference in early April was Dr. Richard M. Pearce, who had recently joined the forces of the Rockefeller Foundation as Director of the Division of Medical Education. He was a man of experience and wisdom. Just when or by whom it was first suggested that it might be helpful to have Dr. Pearce visit Peking, is not clear, but by summer the decision to send him out for a year had been reached. On October 23, 1920, he arrived in Peking with his family.

His first three weeks were spent exploring the administrative situation with Dr. Houghton, Mr. Greene and members of the faculty. This resulted in recommendations from the Administrative Board for faculty participation in academic appointments and educational policy, and for a simplification of the mechanism for dealing with other administrative matters. These recommendations and the budget proposals for 1921-22 were then taken by Dr. Houghton to New York as requested by the chairman of the CMB, Mr. Vincent. The Administrative Board appointed Dr. Pearce to serve as Acting Director during Dr. Houghton's absence.

The day after Dr. Houghton's departure, Dr. Pearce called a special meeting of the Administrative Board at which Dr. Houghton was unanimously recommended to the Trustees for appointment as Director of the College as of January 1, 1921.

The proposals of the Administrative Board which Dr. Houghton carried to New York called for replacement of that Board by two bodies — the Medical Faculty and an Administrative Council, the latter body "to conduct such business as not handled by the Medical Faculty." The organization worked far better than anything that had preceded it. The separation of academic and professional concerns from those of a business and fiscal nature was especially welcomed by the Faculty.

At the outset, the Standing Committees of the Medical Faculty included one on the Hospital. It soon was recognized that most of the business of that committee did not pertain to the Medical Faculty, which thereupon recommended that it be transferred to the Administrative Council. There it stayed until 1927 when the Trustees approved an independent Committee on the Hospital, at the same time that a Committee of Professors was established to deal with appointments to the senior academic ranks and to act in an advisory capacity to the Director on matters of general policy. For the next ten years this was the pattern of the internal administration of the institution — Committee of Professors, Medical Faculty, Committee on the Hospital, Administrative Council.

Building a Faculty

When the China Medical Board assumed full responsibility for the Union Medical College on July 1, 1915, the Medical Faculty consisted almost entirely of the existing "College Teaching Staff." Nineteen persons were then listed covering the fields of anatomy, chemistry, biology, physiology, pathology and bacteriology, surgery, medicine, materia medica, ophthalmology, and gynecology and obstetrics.

When Dr. McLean returned from Peking in the summer of 1916, his first concern was to find suitable personnel for the Premedical School so that it could be opened in the autumn of 1917. He was, however, also already thinking about staff for the preclinical departments in the Medical College and clinicians to strengthen the existing staff of the Hospital. His first recommendation was that of Dr. E. V. Cowdry as Professor of Anatomy. Dr. Cowdry arrived in Peking in September 1918. Dr. Bernard E. Read, a member of the preclinical faculty of the Union Medical College, had been sent to the United States for graduate study in physiological chemistry, from which he returned to serve on the PUMC faculty until 1932 when he resigned the professorship of pharmacology to head the newly organized Lester Institute for Medical Research in Shanghai. Five of the clinicians at the old Union Medical College were soon given new PUMC appointments. Three of these—Dr. J. H. Korns, Dr. J. H. Smyly, and Dr. C. W. Young—continued in the Department of Medicine for the next ten years.

The succeeding years saw the faculty grow in numbers, with a parallel emphasis on quality. When the Trustees met in September 1921 for the Dedication Exercises the medical faculty and staff totaled fifty-seven, a group of men and women whose high professional competence was coupled with an unusual devotion to the institution and its purposes.

Two of the distinguished delegates to the dedication, Dr. A. B. MacCallum, Professor of Biochemistry at McGill University, and Dr. Francis W. Peabody, Professor of Medicine at Harvard (who had been a member of the First China Medical Commission), stayed on for some months and according to the Director "contributed much in the way of counsel, scientific stimulus and practical service during their stay." These were the first of the impressive roster of outstanding men and women who, over the succeeding years, enjoyed service for varying lengths of time as visiting professors in their specialties. In addition, there were visits from traveling medical scientists and teachers who gladly lectured at the PUMC while in Peking and consulted with the faculty. The visiting professors and visitors served to strengthen and develop the specific departments in which they worked. They were also important in helping to dissolve any sense there might be of scientific isolation, and on their return home were able to make the purposes and program of the College better known in the Western world. The visiting professor program facilitated the securing and holding on the staff of valuable men and helped to make the institution a center of scientific interest and activity for the entire Orient. It was also an important factor in the eventual placing of fellows sent abroad for graduate study.

In 1922 Dr. Donald D. Van Slyke was Visiting Professor of Physiological Chemistry for the first trimester of the school year. Not only did he participate in a six-week graduate course in diabetic metabolism, and otherwise enter into the teaching activities of the department, but with Dr. McLean and Dr. Wu Hsien, he tackled what he described at the time as "really a major problem." This was working out the Gibbs-Donnan effect and a complete nomogram for (horse) blood, which Dr. Van Slyke has said was "one of the most important contributions with which I have been associated" for the completion of which he gave credit to the "thirst for work that both my colleagues showed." Dr. McLean himself in retrospect called collaboration in this particular project his own most important contribution to medical research.

Other visiting professors in 1922 were Dr. Ernst Fuchs, the Viennese ophthalmologist; Dr. Reid Hunt, professor of pharmacology at Harvard; Dr. E. C. Dudley, professor emeritus of gynecology at Northwestern University; while Dr. Harry R. Slack of Johns Hopkins Medical School spent that year as head of the department of otolaryngology in the absence on furlough of Dr. Dunlap.

As the years went on, the search for qualities of mind and spirit to meet the challenges of this exciting modern institution set within the walls of the ageless city of Peking was unremitting, for it was on these men and women and those who would join or follow them that success— or failure—would depend.

New York–Peking Relationships

Dr. Pearce was not only a man of wisdom and experience; he was a man of courage and action. Having dealt satisfactorily with the two first items on his agenda—local nomination of the Director, and the reorganization of local administrative control—he turned his attention to the analysis of overall administrative problems between New York and Peking.

He very quickly appreciated the fact that in New York so many different persons had been handling the affairs of the PUMC that there was no consecutive control. Changes in construction and even policy had been decided upon sometimes in ignorance of previous plans. He described the results as frequently "deplorable," making local administration arduous and often putting the director in a difficult position with members of the faculty.

After three months of constant contacts with and study of the various departments of the institution and of those who headed them, he concluded that two things were essential to improve the situation: (1) greater autonomy for the local administration; and (2) immediate delimiting of budgets for the next several years. He pointed out that when it was first decided to establish a Medical School and Hospital, no one had realized that the ultimate plant would of necessity include a premedical school and nurses' training school, two large staff residence compounds, and a physical plant to provide services and utilities which in the United States were available in the community. This had inevitably required more personnel than originally contemplated. Appointment of this personnel and the control of policies had centered largely in the New York office which did not really understand the extent of the interests it was trying to handle. Many detailed matters had to be referred to New York from Peking for decision, involving loss of time and added expense.

Out of his own experience Dr. Pearce forcefully noted: "The management of the institution is hampered in so many ways that without greater autonomy on the part of the local organization it is hardly a worthwhile job. If I had not an abiding interest in the work, and also a desire to assist the Foundation in solving its problems, I would after the first month have asked for a reassignment to duty elsewhere."

Of equal importance in his mind was the setting of budget limits. This was essential if there was to be greater local autonomy as well as an early determination of the final sum necessary in the future for running the institution. The initial open-handed attitude of the Trustees toward capital expenditures for equipment had gone on too long. Department heads did not feel bound to stay within the item for current expenses in their own budgets, but felt free to ask whatever they wished as a matter of capital expenditure going through Mr. Greene directly to the Trustees. Dr. Pearce believed that after the first year of any department its further needs should fall within the annual budget, with decisions to be passed upon by the Director of the PUMC, and not by the Director of the CMB.

Dr. Pearce also called for a review of the salary question with provision for stated increases within grades, thus relieving pressures on department heads and the administration, while also making possible more accurate estimates for the final budget for future years. He considered the cost of the laboratory departments of the medical school, premedical school, and nurses' training school, as "relatively trifling" compared with the expenses of the hospital and physical plant, the limitation of which was, in his opinion, the "really great task" to be faced. This was in line with the separation of educational and administrative activities which had so recently been effected.

While Dr. Pearce was in Peking preparing heads of departments by conferences and suggestion for serious consideration of budget limitations for the years ahead and working out budgets accordingly, Dr. Houghton was in New York conferring with the PUMC Trustees and the CMB on the same subjects, adding the weight of his firsthand knowledge of the situation in Peking to Dr. Pearce's recommendations.

On December 28, 1920, the Trustees took several actions implementing those recommendations: (1) they approved the formal reorganization of the local administration which was already functioning on a provisional basis; (2) adopted a fifteen-point memorandum embodying principles and policies to guide the Faculty and Administrative Council in formulating programs and submitting budget estimates; and (3) appointed Dr. Houghton Director of the PUMC beginning January 1, 1921. With the approval of the first two recommendations, Dr. Houghton was relieved of his previous apprehensions on the difficulties of administering an institution so far from its home base, and promptly accepted the appointment.

The final point in the Trustees' memorandum on programs and budget estimates was a reminder that there were no funds with which to maintain the College "except as these are supplied by sources other than the Board itself" and that The Rockefeller Foundation "with its worldwide responsibilities and opportunities" would have to set a limit to the size of annual appropriations beyond which it would find itself unable to provide funds. With this warning, the budget estimates for 1921-22, which Dr. Houghton had brought from Peking, were sent back for further consideration and reduction.

Dr. Houghton returned to Peking, therefore, to be immediately plunged into the problems of meeting the basic costs of the growing institution, satisfying the desires and aspirations of the lively faculty, and keeping the resultant figures within the limits of what the Trustees and China Medical Board might find reasonable and possible to meet.

The Dedication Exercises

There were still buildings under construction, many departments did not yet have equipment essential for minimal functioning, curriculum planning was of overriding importance as the first medical students — the Class of 1924 — moved toward the years of clinical instruction. The organization of the hospital as an effective teaching facility which also served the community was a new concept which the general public did not always understand. There had been brought together a large and growing staff, international in character and diverse in temperament, who had to learn to live and work together in a new and for many, an alien environment. All this and budgets too would seem to be more than enough for the new Director and his new administration to cope with. But, there was one thing more that made heavy demands on everyone — preparation for a "Formal Opening" in the autumn of 1921.

Tentative discussions on this subject had occurred as early as 1919. As time went on, various suggestions were made which involved much gathering of information, listing of distinguished men of medicine and science from abroad whose presence would make the dedication an event of some international medical significance, exploring the possibility of a concurrent meeting in Peking of the China Medical Missionary Association — these and other proposals absorbed much time, energy and voluminous correspondence. Dr. Pearce was greatly disturbed over the extra work thus thrown upon the staff just as the hospital was being opened and clinical courses were starting. He urged that the occasion should be kept as simple as possible. The proposal to have a meeting of the PUMC Trustees in Peking at the time of the dedication, however, had the warm approval of both Dr. Pearce and Dr. Houghton. Hopefully a study of the institution's problems and needs on the spot would have a beneficial effect on the attitude of the Trustees toward the whole enterprise.

And so the spring and summer of 1921 went by. In New York the Trustees put off as far as possible dealing with matters of substance, while the officers assembled items to be considered at the week-long series of meetings of the Board in Peking in September. One of those items was reconsideration of the 1921-22 operating budget which had been returned to Peking for downward revision. To help the Budget Committee in this painful task, Mr. Edwin R. Embree, Secretary of both the Board of Trustees and the China Medical Board, arrived in Peking in July, with instructions to concentrate on ensuring substantial reductions. His insistence on drastic cuts again raised the specter which Dr. McLean had feared—a willingness to settle for something less than the first-class institution which the founders had said they wanted. Mr. Embree found himself facing strongly determined opposition led by Dr. Pearce, Dr. Houghton and the faculty.

In Peking, budget arguments notwithstanding, the first men patients were moved from the old hospital into the new hospital wards on June 24th. A week later a few women were admitted to "K" Building. Ward by ward, building by building, as the construction gangs left, the equipment went in followed by a staff which had been impatiently awaiting that day. When the Trustees and other distinguished visitors began to arrive early in September, they found a going institution—the stimulating atmosphere of an active staff and eager students.

The invitations to "the dedication of the buildings of the Peking Union Medical College" were for the week of September 15-22. For the eight Trustees who were there, the firsthand study of the institution for whose existence they were responsible, and the sessions of their week-long meeting, adjourned from April 13, 1921, were of greater importance than the formal exercises, speeches and scientific meetings. Beginning September 13 at 10: 15 a. m., through September 21 at 12: 30 p. m., they met daily, except Sunday, in twelve sessions for a total of thirty-six hours, the first four days meeting both morning and afternoon. Dr. Houghton, Mr. Greene and Dr. Pearce sat with the Trustees throughout. Other members of the faculty and administration were called in from time to time for consultation. In addition to specific items requiring action, there was intensive discussion of the institution's program and problems covering a wide range. Dr. Pearce's recommendation for greater local autonomy found a sympathetic hearing and was approved. Four full days were spent on the question of present and future budgets, studying them item by item, department by department, in conference with the head of each department. At the close of these discussions the Trustees approved the budget for 1921-22 in the amount originally requested in December 1920, (Mex.* 1,065,000) after which the officers and members of the CMB and The Rockefeller Foundation who were present, committed themselves to recommend to their boards funds for 1922-23 and 1923-24, to cover budgets of Mex. 1,200,000.

This was a major victory for Dr. Pearce, Dr. Houghton and Mr. Greene, and the other proponents of maintaining the high standards set by the founders. It had been eminently worth while for the PUMC to have this visit from its Trustees.

It was, however, a defeat for Mr. Embree who had faithfully tried to carry out the difficult mission of drastic budget reduction. It would not have been surprising had he viewed the institution and the dedication exercises without much enthusiasm. Quite to the contrary, his informal account of the dedication published in the General Bulletin of the Rockefeller Foundation of October 26, 1921, was the most appreciative and vivid of the many sent back from Peking, as the following excerpts show:

Peking is beautiful in the early autumn. The hutung dust is then less stifling than usual, the open shops present fascinating pictures on all the streets, the itinerant venders and beggars send forth their calls harmoniously, funeral and wedding processions display their most gorgeous designs. Through the clear air the Western Hills stand out green and purple in the distance; and in the foreground rise Coal Hill with its artistic little pagodas, the magnificent gates of the Tartar Wall, the Imperial City with its yellow roofs and, not less conspicuous, the great green roofs of the Yu Wang Fu, the new medical college and hospital.

To see and to dedicate the Peking Union Medical College, scientists and delegates came at this alluring period of the autumn from Japan, from England, Scotland and Ireland, from Java and Korea and the Philippines, from Canada and from France, from the United States and from every important province of China.

The academic procession of these eminent visitors on September 19 was striking in its contrasts. Scientists from the East and from the West marched together in occidental academic costume, passing in slow procession beneath

---

* The fact that the funds of The Rockefeller Foundation were in US dollars (gold) while expenditures in Peking were necessarily in Chinese currency, was always somewhat confusing apart from the question of exchange rates, because over the years a number of different currencies were successively legal tender. The designation *Mex* refers to a silver currency based on the silver content of the Mexican and Spanish dollars which circulated throughout the Far East in the late 19th and early 20th centuries. Other Chinese currency designations which appear in later chapters are: LC (Local Currency); CS (Chinese Silver); FRB (Federal Reserve Bank); CNC (Chinese National Currency); GY (Gold Yuan); JMP (Jen Min P'iao — People's Currency).

the great overhanging roofs of green tile, past modern laboratories and age-old water carts, through rows of students of western medicine and past groups of wondering coolies and ever-present beggars. The street cries of the singing craftsmen merged with the martial rhythm of the new great organ as the column swept slowly into the beautiful temple building which within proved to be a modern auditorium.

While the Trustees wrestled with problems of budgets and policies, a medical conference was in progress with a full program taking advantage of the unusual opportunity to meet and hear the many distinguished visiting scientists.

The high point of the whole week was the actual dedication ceremony at which Dr. Houghton was formally installed as Director, and Mr. John D. Rockefeller, Jr., made the principal address, concluding with these prophetic words, quoted in the Prologue to this chronicle:

Clearly, whatever Western medical science may have to offer China, it will be of little avail to the Chinese people until it is taken over by them and becomes a part of the national life. So we must look forward to the day when most, if not all, of the positions on the Faculty... will be held by Chinese; when the Board of Trustees, while embracing appointees of those bodies which founded the institution, as well as other representatives of Western civilization in China, will include leading Chinese, and when such current support as the institution may need beyond that derived from tuition fees and such endowment as may be set aside by its founders, will be derived from Chinese gifts and governmental subsidies, as is the case with medical institutions of similar rank in other countries of the world. Let us then go forward with one accord towards the attainment of this objective which will make permanent the establishment on Chinese soil of the best in scientific medicine that the world can offer.

In the course of the succeeding weeks most of the visitors went on their way, one or two staying on to give some special lectures at the College, but everyone—students and staff—more than ready to settle down to the work which was the reason they were there.

A heart-warming postscript is the following unsigned letter which appeared in the first issue of the China Medical Journal to be published after the Dedication:

To the Editor, CMJ Dear Sir: These are the days of great suspicion. Everyone who tries to say something is suspected of having an ulterior motive of some sort, surely he must have an axe to grind. Perhaps there will even be those who may suspect that the enclosed is for a reason. It is, but not for that kind of a reason. I happen to have more money in the bank for my work than I know how to spend wisely. That is one reason I do not wish my name to be used.

Some of the brethren in our Association might suggest communism. Another reason is that I do not want any of the readers to suspect that this attempted tribute may be for future reference, They did not give us a chance to say "Thank you" in Peking, so I say it through our Journal.

Sincerely yours,
With my CMMA dues paid up,

....

P. S. I also paid my own travel both ways and board bill in Peking. Have I disarmed everybody?

The biggest impression made upon me while in Peking attending the formal opening of Peking Union Medical College was not made by the physical plant. When I came to China I was sent into the back country and have never become familiar with the stringent requirements for a modern medical school and large hospital. Those who know more about these things and about art and architecture than I do, probably had a hard time to restrain their enthusiasm.

Ignorance saved me. But I noted that there was ample ground for every building and inside these buildings everybody seemed to have plenty of room in which to work. The buildings are so clean and well-lighted and substantial. Just to be in and out of them day after day put new spring into my legs and ginger into the day's program. But the physical plant, magnificent as it is, made an impression of secondary importance upon me.

This is what constantly impressed me. The spirit of the men I met there. Like many others, I have known Mr. Greene and Dr. Houghton for years. I found them just the same splendid, clear thinking men we all know them to be. They gave me no new surprises and I centered my attention upon the new-comers—members of the faculty just out from home, members of the Board of Trustees of the China Medical Board, and particularly Mr. John D. Rockefeller, Jr., himself. Without intruding, I made it my business to meet them. This was easy because they are democratic citizens. I also attended every meeting I could to hear what they had to say. The end of every day found me dead tired, but happy. I say happy because I believe these men are trying to serve China just as truly as I am. Before I reached Peking I had heard occasional disquieting words about the school and how it might exert an influence not fully in line with the present needs in medical education in China. I can only wish that those whose minds are ill at ease still will make it a point to read the addresses delivered by Mr. Rockefeller, Dr. Vincent, Mr. Greene, Dr. Houghton and others during the dedicatory week. My feelings are pretty well case hardened, but I was stirred to the depths of my heart by the fine spirit each one of them manifested. This new advance in medical education is in good hands.

It was a revelation to me to learn of the difficulties they encountered in delay and cost of construction because of the war. They are exercising great care in their choice of personnel. I am tempted to become personal and pay tribute to some of the men I met there during my stay, splendid men whose leadership I shall accept gladly. Of course, their standards are high, higher than any we have in China today but not a bit higher than we ought to have. Had they been lower I would have been able to rub off only three layers of rust during my short stay instead of the nine or ten which my medical mind experienced. For one, I hope to avail myself of their post-graduate courses whenever I get an opportunity. It will be a great thing for me to be able to take my dull axe to a fine grindstone in China without having to go abroad each time only to dissipate much of my energy in speech making and housekeeping. I understand they are quite prepared to "flunk" any missionary who does not do good work. That's the place for me!

Only one defect in the program of the opening revealed itself and became more acute with each day. Toward the end of the week some of us discussed it together but there did not seem to be anything we could do. The talking was all done from their side of the fence. Of course, the officials of the China Medical Board and the distinguished guests all could make better speeches than any of us from the back woods of China, but having this continue day after day really became a painful experience. I was tempted a dozen times to stand right up in meeting and shout out what was on my heart to say, "We're glad you're here!" There was not a single chance for us to say openly the thanks we felt. Somebody should have done it spontaneously for the feeling was real and widespread among the China delegates. Now, if you don't mind my saying so, I allowed my bottled-up feelings to express themselves in a prayer of thanksgiving for what Mr. Rockefeller and his associates in this enterprise had achieved and of supplication that the whole undertaking might be of great blessing to China and the world.

Peking Union Medical College, rechristened, enlarged, strengthened, had a most auspicious opening. Perhaps the contrast is too great to put it this way, but we on both sides of the Pacific sacrificed together to make possible and then enjoy this wonderful dedication week. It was not easy for those of us in China to drop our work for so long a time as this with travel required. But those coming from abroad, Mr. Rockefeller, the President Elect of the American Medical Association, and the many distinguished persons from other countries certainly found it no easier. Having been at Peking, I shall never be so easily satisfied in the future with low standards and careless work.

May the highest expectations of the founders of the institution be realized through the years to come. And in this realization, each one of us may have a small but vital share through our sympathy and support.

Chapter III

YEARS OF GROWTH

1922-1936

THE YEARS following the Dedication were years of political unrest and frequent military disturbances. Collaboration of the Kuomintang with the Soviet Union and the Chinese Communist Party; the death in Peking on March 12, 1925, of Dr. Sun Yat-sen;[*] and the establishment in Canton on July 1, 1925, of a "National Government;" were followed by the historic Northward Expedition launched by Chiang Kai-shek in the summer of 1926. The sweep north went so rapidly that it got badly out of hand, with tragic excesses of the victorious army against Chinese and "foreigner" alike, leaving death and devastation and fear of what a China under Kuomintang control might become. The warlords who had kept the country in turmoil since 1911 had been bad; would the Kuomintang be worse? During 1927 and much of 1928, there was active dissension between the radicals and the moderates in the Nationalist movement, with rival capitals in Hankow and Nanking, but by November 1927 the radical Hankow government had collapsed, the Nanking Government expelled Soviet consuls and commercial agents from the country, and the Kuomintang armies started their northward trek once more. It was June 1928

---

[*] A patient in the PUMC Hospital during his final illness, Dr. Sun died in his own home where he had been taken a few days before his death. A Christian funeral service was held in the PUMC Auditorium, following which his body was at the Pi Yun Ssu Temple in the Western Hills until 1929, when it was ceremoniously removed to the Mausoleum built on the side of Purple Mountain in Nanking.

when Peking, after years at the mercy of warring generals and cliques, fell to the Nationalists and was renamed Peiping (interpreted by some as "Northern Peace" and by others as "Pacified North"). On October 10 of that year, Chiang Kai-shek assumed the chairmanship of the National Government at its chosen capital, Nanking.

What of the PUMC during these troublesome years? The hospital and out-patient department were filled to capacity and clamoring for room to expand their services—gratifying evidence of the acceptance of PUMC clinical standards by the Peking populace.

The first class of students graduated in June 1924—three doctors, one nurse—the student body meanwhile steadily building up in quality as well as numbers. Although most students were too absorbed in their professional studies to be drawn into political activities (how strange that sounds in 1970), disruptive action in other schools and colleges in Peking caused the abrupt termination of the academic year before the June examinations which were held over until autumn. The faculty and administration congratulated themselves that nothing more serious had happened.

The faculty, rounded out and with a deliberate increase in Chinese and a corresponding decrease in Westerners, was active in many ways. Experience and study led to modifications of the over-rigid curriculum of the early years. The program of intensive courses for graduate physicians was set in motion, and a wide variety of research was carried on. This included the groundwork for the noted paleontological studies of Dr. Davidson Black (see p. 84), and the important investigation into the Chinese medicinal plant *Ma-Huang* by Drs. B. E. Read, Carl Schmidt, and K. K. Chen. This came about in the course of a systematic study of the Chinese pharmacopeia and led to the isolation of the alkaloid ephedrine, which became widely used by otolaryngologists in the West until the development of the synthetic products now commonly used. During Dr. Houghton's furlough in 1924-1925 Dr. W. S. Carter, Associate Director of the Division of Medical Education of The Rockefeller Foundation, was Acting Director in Peking.

In September 1925, Dr. John B. Grant, who for many years was a member of the PUMC faculty on loan from the International Health Division of The Rockefeller Foundation, stimulated the establishment by the Peking municipal authorities of a demonstration health center in a ward of the city not far from the PUMC. This center, known as the

First Health Station, was a pilot project in developing health services for the people. For the College it provided facilities for practical training in the public health field comparable to those which the students had in the hospital for their clinical studies. The importance of such controlled practice facilities in public health is now generally accepted, but when the First Health Station was organized in Peking this was a decided departure from the type of public health teaching in most medical schools in the United States and Europe, and was the only thing of its kind in China. The pattern thus set was followed by other Chinese medical schools and the use of health centers in community medical care became a part of the program of the Ministry of Health when it was established by the Nationalist Government in 1929. In an article about the new Ministry, the Vice-Minister wrote that the influence of the Health Demonstration Station in Peking on recent developments of public health in China could "hardly be over-estimated." Indeed, the Ministry of Health drew heavily on the personnel of the First Health Station to staff its own new programs.

The establishment of the First Health Station was equally important to the nurses. Ample opportunity for practical work in the hospital wards and clinics had been provided as a part of the educational program, the routine care of patients in the hospital being carried *not* by student nurses but by staff nurses, a progressive concept not then accepted by many leading hospitals in the United States. Now it would be possible to extend this educational approach to public health nursing using this pioneering practice field.

In the meantime by setting standards of admission and academic performance at a high level, Miss Wolf and her nursing colleagues were demonstrating to a growing number of intelligent young Chinese women that nursing was a profession in which they could find satisfaction. Registration of the school by the Regents of the University of the State of New York having been secured in April 1923, the Trustees changed its name from the *Training School for Nurses* to the *School of Nursing*, clearly acknowledging acceptance of the modern concept of nursing education on a professional level. When the following year Miss Wolf was offered reappointment as Superintendent of Nurses, the Trustees added to her title that of Dean of the School of Nursing, thereby strengthening the school's professional status still further. Miss Wolf did not find it possible to accept reappointment, but she could leave Peking feeling that the foundations had been wisely and surely laid.

Miss Ruth Ingram succeeded to the post bringing not only the requisite professional and administrative qualifications but, having been born in China, an intimate knowledge of the Chinese people and fluency in the Chinese language, invaluable assets in those years of military and political turmoil. In 1929 Miss Ingram returned to the United States, and was succeeded temporarily by Miss Erma B. Taylor, a member of the Nursing Faculty, who served until November 1930 when, on recommendation of Mary Beard and Annie W. Goodrich, the leading nursing educators in the United States at that time, Miss Gertrude E. Hodgman arrived in Peking to assume the Deanship.

Incorporation and Endowment of China Medical Board

At the same time, things were happening in New York which had an important bearing on the College and its future. The Rockefeller Foundation in 1924 as it rounded out its first decade of diverse and rapidly expanding activities decided to review its own policies and administrative structure, especially in relation to the other Rockefeller-sponsored Boards—the General Education Board, the International Education Board, and the Laura Spelman Rockefeller Memorial. The China Medical Board as a specialized agency in the Foundation came within the scope of this review.

The composition of the committee of three named to undertake this formidable task—Mr. John G. Agar, Mr. Raymond B. Fosdick, and Dr. Simon Flexner—gave assurance that as far as the CMB and the PUMC were concerned, each of the three was on familiar ground. Mr. Agar and Mr. Fosdick had both been members of the CMB and its Executive Committee, while Dr. Flexner had been a member of the second China Medical Commission in 1915, an "original member" of both the CMB and the PUMC Trustees, and was currently a member of the Executive Committee of the latter body. Their first recommendation affecting specifically the CMB and the PUMC called for the transfer of the functions of the CMB to the Division of Medical Education of The Rockefeller Foundation, disbanding the CMB as a specialized organ of the Foundation, eventual transfer of the Peking property to the College, and organization of a new American corporation (the CMB Inc.) to receive from The

Rockefeller Foundation sufficient funds to yield the income needed by the institution, thus relieving the Foundation of further responsibility for its maintenance. This far-reaching recommendation was made in November 1926, accepted by the Foundation Trustees on February 23, 1927, and on April 1, 1927, the functions of the China Medical Board were transferred to the Division of Medical Education of which Dr. Richard M. Pearce was Director. For the next eighteen months, all matters concerning the PUMC, such as appointments and budgets, are recorded in the Minutes of the regular meetings of the Trustees of The Rockefeller Foundation.

On May 23, 1928, the Trustees of The Rockefeller Foundation took a series of actions of major importance affecting the organization of the Foundation and its associated boards. These included an action for which the College's friends in the Foundation and in China had been anxiously hoping—appropriation to the China Medical Board, Inc., as soon as its legal incorporation should be accomplished, of US$12,000,000, the income designated for the support of first, the PUMC and second, similar institutions in the Far East and in the United States (the wisdom of this second "escape" clause is evident today in the wide-ranging program developed by China Medical Board, Inc. since 1951). Recognizing that the income on $12,000,000 would be insufficient to cover current PUMC budgets the Foundation also undertook to supplement that income for the five years between 1928 and 1933 to a total of $1,500,000, in diminishing annual grants, and to review the situation at the end of the five-year period.

It should not be forgotten that these discussions and actions, designed to set the enterprise on a sound and independent basis, were going on against the background of turmoil described at the beginning of this chapter. The wonder is that the founders did not throw up their hands in dismay, decide to cut their losses by abandoning the project, and look for some more stable field of operations. Instead, with an unparalleled act of faith they confirmed their commitment to the objective of "making permanent the establishment on Chinese soil of the best in scientific medicine that the world can offer" and on November 9, 1928, turned over to China Medical Board, Inc., $12,000,000 as endowment.

Changing the Guard

The momentous discussions and actions in New York were reflected in various ways in Peking. The changes in administrative leadership of the College at the beginning of 1928, though not a direct result of what was happening at the home base, were certainly related to it.

Dr. Houghton had long planned that when the institution was well on its feet he would seek to establish himself in the United States so as to avoid the family separations otherwise entailed in the education of his five children. When in the summer of 1927 he was offered the Deanship of the Medical School of the University of Iowa, he felt free to give this serious consideration, confident that he would leave the PUMC on sound educational and administrative foundations and with its future assured by the plans being developed in New York for incorporating and endowing the China Medical Board. After careful consideration and a quick trip for conferences in Iowa City and New York, Dr. Houghton returned to Peking and submitted his resignation as Director effective January 31, 1928.

During the year 1927-1928, Dr. F. C. Yen, Dean of the Hsiang-Ya Medical School which had temporarily closed as a result of the disturbed political and military situation in Hunan Province, was serving as Vice Director of the College, a post recently created by the Trustees in the hope that a Chinese in this position might meet anticipated Chinese educational regulations. Since Dr. Yen's appointment was only for the short term before his expected return to Hsiang-Ya, it was necessary to take early steps for the appointment of a successor to him as well as to Dr. Houghton. The Committee of Professors which was responsible for recommending candidates for the offices of Director and Vice Director made two unanimous recommendations: Dr. Liu Jui-heng (then serving as professor of surgery) as Vice Director, concurrently with his appointment as Medical Superintendent of the Hospital; and Mr. Roger S. Greene as Acting Director from January 1, 1928. On December 28, 1927, Dr. Houghton left Peking with his family, bringing to a close eleven and a half years of uninterrupted service to The Rockefeller Foundation, the China Medical Board, and the Peking Union Medical College whose Director he had been for seven years.

As could be expected, the transition to Mr. Greene's directorship was smooth. For years he and Dr. Houghton had worked in such close cooperation that each could pick up the other's particular responsibilities easily when necessary. Indeed, as one goes through the files and the official records it is often difficult to determine when either of them was acting as an officer of the CMB or of the PUMC. The fact is that both men were completely dedicated to the development of the College and were ready to respond to whatever demands were put upon them.

Registration with the Ministry of Education and Reorganizing the Board of Trustees

On January 1, 1928, when Mr. Greene took up the post of Acting Director, the institution was a going concern. While involving himself fully in the normally recurring questions of staff, students, academic and scientific programs, and hospital service, he was accordingly able to devote much time to laying the groundwork locally for the reorganization of the basic structure of the College which was corollary to the major changes in The Rockefeller Foundation and China Medical Board described above.

His concurrent post as Vice President in the Far East of The Rockefeller Foundation kept him informed on the developing situation in New York. His broad acquaintance among leaders, Chinese and Western, in education and government gave him an insight into the momentous changes that were taking place in China so that when Peking fell to the Nationalists in June 1928, he was prepared for the fact that this foreshadowed effective control by the Nanking government. The Ministry of Education had, indeed, already promulgated its first regulations affecting institutions of higher learning which included the requirement that the president—or director—be Chinese and that a majority of the Trustees should be Chinese.

In the meantime, the amendment of the provisional charter by the Regents of the University of the State of New York at the request of the PUMC Trustees, had made that body self-perpetuating, thus providing machinery for orderly revamping of the Board of Trustees should government regulations make this desirable or necessary.

Early in 1929, Mr. Greene went to New York at the suggestion of the CMB to attend the spring meetings of the Board and of the PUMC Trustees. In preparation for his trip, Mr. Greene had conferred at length on all these questions with the Committee of Professors as well as with the Minister of Education of the Nationalist Government in Nanking. He took with him a recommendation from the professors that if the Trustees should decide upon registration of the College under the new regulations of the Ministry of Education, Dr. J. Heng Liu be named Director, and

Mr. Greene, Vice Director. The Ministry had indicated that Dr. Liu would be acceptable as Director, a proposal which Mr. Greene warmly favored. The precise functions to be discharged by the Director would depend on whether Dr. Liu returned to Peking or continued on leave of absence in Nanking, where he had been serving as head of the newly formed Ministry of Health since 1928. Mr. Greene was confident that some satisfactory arrangement could be worked out. He himself would be happy to serve as Vice Director under Dr. Liu.

Before the Annual Meeting of the PUMC Trustees in New York on April 10, 1929, each Trustee received a long and detailed memorandum, with arguments for and against four possible courses of action. All but two members of the Board were present at this meeting. The morning session was devoted to normal business—reports and budgets. It was after lunch that the item in the Docket headed REGISTRATION OF THE COLLEGE AND REQUIREMENTS OF THE CHINESE GOVERNMENT was taken up. How long the discussion lasted, the Minutes do not record but it resulted in the adoption of a resolution stating "the sense of this Board that the most appropriate means of meeting the requirements of the Chinese Government will be through changes in membership of the present Board of Trustees." One by one, the Trustees went through the formal motions of submitting their resignations and voting on their successors. The stilted language of the next five pages of Minutes does not dim the vivid picture of the drama taking place. When the meeting opened, there were thirteen Trustees in office—one a Chinese; by the close of the meeting, five more Chinese had been elected, the process of securing a majority being completed at the first meeting of the new Board in Peking on July 5, 1929, when one resignation received too late for the April meeting was accepted and a Chinese elected to fill this place.

The roll of Chinese Trustees was distinguished: Dr. Alfred Sao-ke Sze, Dr. Chang Po-ling, Dr. C. C. Wu, Dr. J. Heng Liu, Dr. Hu Shih, Dr. Y. T. Tsur, Dr. Wong Wen-hao. It needed to be, for the men whom they replaced were Dr. Thomas Cochrane, Dr. Simon Flexner, Dr. Frank Mason North, Mr. John D. Rockefeller, Jr., Dr. H. H. Weir, and Dr. William H. Welch, each one of whom had played a significant part in the founding and building of the institution which they were now turning over, as originally planned, to Chinese administrative control.

The election of a Board, the majority of whom were resident in China, meant that thereafter meetings would of necessity be in that country. Pending the first meeting in Peking when the newly-elected Trustees could themselves act, interim appointments of officers were approved: Mr. Greene and Dr. Chang Po-ling, Chairman and Vice Chairman respectively; Dr. J. Heng Liu, Director; Mr. Greene, Vice Director. It was agreed that for the time being the offices of the Secretary and the Treasurer should remain in New York, the College thus continuing to profit during the transitional period of new relationships between the Trustees and the CMB by the experienced services and advice of Miss Eggleston and Mr. Myers, who had for so long served the Trustees in these capacities.

When next the Trustees met, it was in Peking where the new Board took up its responsibilities on July 5, 1929. Writing to Dr. Pearce about that meeting, Mr. Greene reported that he was "well pleased with our new Board" and believed that it would function as efficiently as the previous one. "The members are certainly much interested and they will soon be better informed and therefore better able to help the officers in dealing with local problems." Dr. Y. T. Tsur was elected Chairman, Dr. Chang Po-ling re-elected Vice Chairman; Miss Eggleston and Mr. Myers were confirmed as Secretary and Treasurer in New York, with an Assistant Secretary, Miss Alberta Worthington, to perform the necessary functions of the secretary in Peking. An Executive Committee of Trustees resident in North China provided for effective handling of business between meetings of the full Board. Dr. Liu[*] and Mr. Greene were confirmed in their administrative posts. The officers were instructed to take immediate steps to secure the registration of the College with the Ministry of Education; a Constitution and By-laws conforming to the government regulations were approved; the suggestion of their predecessors for the establishment of an Advisory Committee in the United States made up of former Trustees—Dr. James L. Barton, Dr. Arthur J. Brown, Dr. Simon Flexner, Dr. Paul Monroe, Mr. John D. Rockefeller, Jr., Mr. George E. Vincent, and Dr. Richard M. Pearce—was warmly endorsed and a vote of appreciation extended to all members of the former Board of Trustees for past services to the College. The new Board was in business!

---

* He had agreed to accept the title of Director with the understanding that he would continue on leave of absence while serving as head of the National Health Administration in Nanking.

Their education as Trustees proceeded apace. Meetings of the Executive Committee on July 23, August 22, October 11, November 27, and December 30, show how much it meant to Mr. Greene to have these men readily available for consultation. Miss Eggleston, out of her long experience, kept a watchful and helpful eye on the dockets and minutes sent to her from Peking, forewarning Mr. Greene and the Assistant Secretary of meetings scheduled in New York with which the Peking calendar must be coordinated, calling attention to the importance of not overstepping limitations of authority prescribed in the By-laws, while at the same time continuing to handle contacts with prospective staff members, arrangements for travel for families on furlough, shepherding fellowship-holders through their problems, great or small, in a strange land, and countless other services to the College.

The application for registration could not be submitted before September since the Ministry of Education would only send its examiners to inspect the institution while it was in session. Before the fall term opened, however, Mr. Greene learned to his dismay that the Ministry had promulgated new regulations raising the number of Chinese Trustees required to a *two-thirds* majority. This was not a "minor change" such as the Executive Committee had been authorized to deal with, but would necessitate action by the whole Board of Trustees amending the Constitution adopted on July 5, 1929, which followed the original requirement of a simple majority. In addition, Mr. Greene was informed that to conform with the latest regulations, the By-laws must be amended to provide that senior administrative officers be appointed by the Director rather than by the Trustees.

These new developments he discussed with Dr. Tsur, Chairman of the Board. Dr. Tsur was reluctant to increase the number of Chinese Trustees at the cost of resignations of any more non-Chinese members. On the other hand, enlarging the Board involved amending its charter from the Regents of the University of the State of New York, a time-consuming process just when it was important for the continuance of the College and for the recognition of its graduates that registration should not be too long deferred.

After consultation with all available Trustees, correspondence with Dr. Pearce, Mr. Vincent and the Advisory Committee in the United States, and with the understanding concurrence of two valued long-time members of the Board, it was decided that two steps should be taken: (1) Dr. Paul Monroe and Mr. F. H. Hawkins would resign as Trustees, to be replaced by two Chinese, thus securing without delay the two-thirds majority necessary for registration; (2) early application should be made to the Regents for an amendment of the provisional charter increasing the number of Trustees from thirteen to not more than twenty-five, in the expectation that Dr. Monroe and Mr. Hawkins would be re-elected to the Board along with enough additional Chinese to maintain the required two-thirds majority.

On February 8, 1930, a special meeting of the Board of Trustees in Shanghai approved these steps, amended the Constitution and By-laws as required, and requested the Regents simultaneously to change the name of the institution to the Peiping Union Medical College to conform with the recent change in name of the city. The two new Chinese Trustees were of the same high calibre as those previously elected: Dr. W. W. Yen and Mr. Sohtsu G. King. On May 21, 1930, the Ministry of Education approved the registration of the College.

Budgets and Exchange Rates

Mr. Greene had been so closely involved in all the discussions in New York preceding the incorporation and endowment of the China Medical Board, that he had a clear understanding of the two-fold implications in terms of the College budget: (1) within the limits of the China Medical Board's annual endowment income plus the supplementary annual grants pledged by The Rockefeller Foundation for the five years ending June 1933, the institution was in the unusual and enviable position of absolute financial security; (2) the explicit statement by The Rockefeller Foundation that during this five-year period "no other appropriations... would in any circumstances be made by The Rockefeller Foundation for the purposes of the Board or towards the official budget of the Peking Union Medical College" closed that door firmly to any early expansion of existing programs or addition of others.

It was not always easy to convince department heads that no matter how strong an argument could be made for an urgent need or challenging opportunity, The Rockefeller Foundation meant what it had said. A case in point was the question of the woeful inadequacy of the space allotted to the Library—reading room for not more than six persons at work at the same time! The Library had been supplied at the outset with an outstanding collection of bound periodicals and its budget for current purchases and subscriptions was respectable, but for all who wanted to see the Library *used*, its physical needs continued to be a very live issue.

As the institution grew, this situation became more and more acute. All were agreed that the ideal would be a new building, specifically planned for the Library. Failing that, Laura Spelman House, the original nurses' dormitory, might be adapted for library use, since the recent completion of the new and larger Oliver Jones Hall now cared for housing most of the nurses. Some of the professors felt that a strong case could and should be made for a new building, Foundation policy notwithstanding, with Laura Spelman House reserved for expansion of the hospital. It fell to Mr. Greene (who personally would have liked to see both a new library building and a larger hospital) to emphasize the expressed policy of the Foundation not to grant further capital funds to the College at that time, and to call attention to the fact that any increase in hospital beds would mean increased operating costs which the limitations of the budget could not meet. In the end, the transfer of the library to Laura Spelman House was accepted by the professors as a "temporary measure" but they went on record as considering an adequate and especially designed building for the Library to be an essential part of the physical equipment of the College, and urged that as soon as feasible an application be made to the Foundation for the necessary funds for its construction. As it turned out, Laura Spelman House proved so well-adapted for the purposes of the library that the question of a new building was never raised again.

The fact that Mr. Greene so meticulously held the line on not asking the Foundation for grants over and above those promised for the five-year period did not mean that he accepted the idea of a static establishment. Far from it. Because these annual supplementary grants were on a decreasing basis he was increasingly concerned with how to provide for the normal growth which any healthy institution must have. Every possible economy was effected, beginning with his own and other administrative offices. Ways to raise the level of local hospital income were sought. Long-range plans were made for a considerable reduction of foreign staff, with replacements by Chinese whose salaries would be on the new local currency scale.

With this approach and in spite of the inevitable pressures from the faculty for increased budgets, the budget for 1930-31 was held to a net figure of Mex. $1,700,000--US$850,000 at the accustomed rate of 2 to 1, an amount covered by the assured endowment income of the CMB plus the Foundation grant for that year. Mr. Greene was proud of the fact that without exceeding the amount available the budget actually provided for a considerable increase in activity, and was less than Mex. $5,000 more than the budget for the previous year.

The meeting of the CMB on April 17, 1930, where the request from the PUMC Trustees for an appropriation to cover this budget was considered, was the first since the death on February 16 of Dr. Richard M. Pearce. Although CMB income had not been directly affected by the stock market crash of October 29, 1929 and its aftermath, the recent financial debacle undoubtedly helped to induce caution when the three surviving members of the Board took up the budget request. After recording their understanding (which was actually erroneous) that the decreasing annual grants from the Rockefeller Foundation assumed that College budgets would be reduced year by year, they returned the 1930-31 budget to the College for revision to a total not more than that for 1929-30, softening the action by expressing willingness to reconsider it at some later date if more detailed information should make this desirable, and in the meantime appropriating a sum equal to one-half the 1929-30 budget to cover operation for the first six months. Two elections at this meeting to fill vacancies on the Board were important to the College: Mr. George E. Vincent and Mr. John D. Rockefeller, 3rd, the latter being also elected Secretary of the CMB.

Had Dr. Pearce been alive to attend this meeting, his intimate knowledge of all that was involved in the development of the College and his understanding of the details of the budget might have reassured the cautious Board members that here was no unreasonable extravagance but rather a careful and thrifty stretching of available resources so as to increase the effectiveness of the institution. As it was, it did not occur to these members of the CMB how seriously disturbing their action might be to the PUMC Trustees and Acting Director to whom the responsibility of internal administration had so recently been entrusted.

When news of the CMB action reached Mr. Greene by cable, he was not only surprised, but in his own words "profoundly disappointed." This was in the days before trans-Pacific air mail. No explanatory letter could be expected before the middle of May. He, therefore, immediately addressed a cable of strong protest to Mr. Fosdick, who had been the prime mover in the incorporation of the CMB and in the setting up of the resultant pattern of supplementary grants by the Foundation. Mr. Fosdick had in the meantime left for Europe and Mr. Greene's cable was turned over to Mr. Vincent as the member most familiar with PUMC affairs. There followed an extended discussion by cable and letter in which Mr. Greene, Mr. Vincent, Mr. Rockefeller, 3rd, and Miss Eggleston all took part. On June 12, 1930, after Mr. Fosdick's return he met with Mr. Vincent and Mr. Rockefeller, 3rd, to reconsider the CMB budget actions in the light of the objections and explanations put forward by Mr. Greene. They evidently found these convincing, for they amended the April action on the budget to provide the full $850,000 requested, and in addition agreed that in the future any unexpended balances in the operating budget at the end of a year should become the property of the PUMC Trustees, to be used for the Corporate Purposes of the College.

Mr. Greene had made his point, an important one especially in terms of developing a responsible Board of Trustees, but one can see in this correspondence and in the formal language of the Minutes signs that the incorporation and endowment had not altogether solved earlier problems but had indeed initiated a new set of stresses and strains, of misunderstandings and cross-purposes, which were increasingly to disturb relationships between New York and Peking.

Mr. Greene as a layman without previous medical experience frequently turned to the Committee of Professors as a group and to individual faculty members personally for advice and suggestions on matters of policy, which gave him a valued sense of support as the College moved steadily ahead toward its goal of *quality*—Chinese governmental pressures for *quantity* production notwithstanding. He sought constantly for ways of meeting departmental needs in personnel, equipment and physical facilities. He wrestled with the budget—and when in the spring of 1929 the rate of exchange began to slip from the long-established norm of one U.S. dollar (gold) to two dollars of local silver currency (Mex), he studied the implications of this new situation intensively. First the rate went to 2.40 to 1; early in 1930 it was in the vicinity of three to one and by mid-June 1930, there was near panic as the rates approached four to one.

The College budget expressed in Mex dollars at two to one was increasingly unrealistic. In the matter of salaries it became necessary in the spring of 1930 for the Trustees to approve salary payments in gold for foreign staff members, leaving it to each one to handle his own exchange transactions. To the Chinese staff, although living on a Chinese scale, this seemed an injustice since rising living costs made their Mex. Salaries less and less adequate. The auditors who had originally approved the accounting system set up by the comptroller of The Rockefeller Foundation which routinely converted all gold expenditures into silver at two to one, began to challenge its soundness under existing conditions.

As these problems mounted, it was a source of great strength to the administrative officers that the Trustees were near at hand and available for frequent informal as well as formal consultation. Personal experience with the rising cost of living made them very ready to set in motion a restudy of the salary scale. They recognized the artificiality of the existing budget and accounting procedures and looked to Mr. Greene and the financial officers of the College and of the CMB to make recommendations for changes that would bring them in line with reality.

At the same time, Mr. Greene kept a steady flow of information going to New York. Without waiting until he and the Trustees were ready to suggest a solution, he sent to Mr. Vincent, Mr. Rockefeller, 3rd, President Mason of The Rockefeller Foundation, and others, memoranda which in historical perspective are convincing expositions of the factors involved — but often so lengthy that it is not surprising if men whose desks were already piled high with other equally weighty business pressed by equally ardent advocates, sometimes pushed them aside without as sympathetic a response as they deserved.

The operating budget for 1931-32 was the first to be expressed realistically in US dollars and Chinese silver currency, bringing to the forefront the matter of rates of exchange between these two currencies which was of such great importance in determining the financial commitment of the China Medical Board, Inc. to the support of the PUMC. Without going into the details of preparing that budget, its adoption by the Trustees, and its approval by the CMB, it is sufficient to say that it was at this point that differences of opinion as to policy and procedure in the handling of exchange began to show themselves between New York and Peking in general, and Mr. Rockefeller, 3rd and Mr. Greene in particular.

Mr. Greene had expected to take this budget to New York in the late winter of 1931, but circumstances in Peking and in New York led to an agreement that rather than going at that time, he should plan a visit around the middle of May 1932. This would allow him to take part in the budget-making for 1932-33, present the budget to the PUMC Trustees at their Annual Meeting on April 13, and bring to the CMB at a special meeting in June a firsthand report of the Trustees' requests.

The fact that he would not have to leave before the spring of 1932 was a great relief to Mr. Greene—there was much to do in Peking. In the summer of 1931, at the request of the National Government, a medical unit had been sent to Nanchang in Kiangsi Province to help in the care of soldiers wounded in the campaign against the communists. This was followed in late September by a request from the National Flood Relief Commission for cooperation in the prevention and treatment of sickness during the autumn and winter among the many refugees from the disastrous summer floods in the Yangtze valley, especially in the Hankow-Wuchang region. Doctors, nurses and students joined in volunteering for this service for varying periods of time, the last unit returning to Peking early in January 1932.

These were not the first nor the last such calls on the College for professional assistance in times of disaster, each occasion seriously disrupting the regular teaching and hospital work of the institution, and often requiring difficult and delicate administrative decisions affecting the institution's relationships with the national health and educational authorities. The fact that the head of the National Health Administration was Dr. J. Heng Liu, Director of the College on leave of absence to serve in that post, and that Dr. John B. Grant, the College's professor of hygiene and public health, was a key adviser of Dr. Liu, sometimes made these decisions easier; at other times, their very closeness to the institution made them expect more in the way of automatic acquiescence than Mr. Greene and other members of the faculty felt was justified. In any case, Mr. Greene was glad that he could see the flood relief participation carried to a satisfactory conclusion.

The political pot was also boiling again. The early summer had seen a group of Kuomintang dissidents in Canton, headed by Wang Ching-wei, Tang Shao-yi and Chen Chi-tang, launching a plot to overthrow the Nanking government headed by Chiang Kai-shek. In June, Chiang took personal command of the "Communist-Suppression Campaign" aimed at the dissidents. In mid-September, Japanese troops occupied Mukden in a surprise attack; by the end of the month other important cities in Manchuria fell into Japanese hands in rapid succession. The Japanese threat resulted in peace negotiations between representatives of the Nanking and Canton faction in Shanghai in late October. On December 15, Chiang Kai-shek once again retired in the interest of party unity, and on January 1, 1932, the reorganized National Government was inaugurated with Lin Sen as Chairman of the government and Sun Fo, President of the Executive Yuan. In less than a month, Japanese troops were fighting in Shanghai and the National Government moved to Loyang, Honan, in the face of a threatened Japanese attack on Nanking.

March 1932 saw the creation of the Japanese puppet state of "Manchukuo" with Henry Pu Yi—the emperor who as a boy had abdicated the Chinese Imperial throne in 1912—as its Chief Executive, and the arrival in China of the League of Nations' Lytton Commission of Enquiry to investigate the "Mukden Incident."

In April, a National Emergency Conference in Loyang decided on prolonged resistance to Japanese aggression, a National Military Council having already been created with Chiang Kai-shek as Chairman. In the meantime, Chinese communists had taken advantage of the Manchurian situation to resume fighting in Central China, and Chiang Kai-shek headed a campaign from Hankow which by the end of the year succeeded in dislodging them from their strongholds in that part of the country.

On May 1, the National Government and the Japanese agreed on an armistice which brought the Japanese attack on Shanghai to an end. For the moment overt Japanese threats had ceased, and with the rout of the communists by Chiang Kai-shek, it seemed safe for the government to return to Nanking from Loyang at the beginning of December, and to open the third plenary session of the Central Executive Committee of the Kuomintang on December 16. It was less than a month later that Japanese troops from outside the Great Wall took Shanhaikuan. For the next five months North China was the Japanese target, with advances toward Peking and Tientsin, the hostilities again ending in a Sino-Japanese Armistice signed on March 31, 1933 in Tangku.

The budget for 1932-33, which Mr. Greene took to New York the end of April 1932 after it had been approved by the Trustees, worked out to a total of US$709,329—the exact amount of appropriations actually made for 1931-32. It was gratifying to be able to report to the CMB that while there was actually a proposed increase in gross expenditures of about US$15,000, this was offset by hospital income which had been steadily increasing in spite of political unrest and commercial depression. The local currency budget showed an increase of some Mex. 200,000, which was well covered by the conservative exchange rate of 4.30 to 1.

Mr. Greene's two and a half months in the United States were filled with numerous conferences and discussions with the officers of the Board, especially with Mr. Rockefeller, 3rd, Secretary of the CMB and a member of the Finance Committee. This was the first formal relationship of Mr. Rockefeller to any of the Rockefeller-related boards, a responsibility which he took seriously. Having addressed himself specifically to the problems of financing and exchange about which he and Mr. Greene had already expressed differences of opinion by correspondence in recent months, this was the major subject of discussion when they met in New York. Their first conferences proved difficult. Mr. Greene, Director of the CMB as well as Acting Director of the PUMC, felt himself senior in point of authority as well as years (Mr. Rockefeller was twenty-five). Mr. Rockefeller, Secretary of the Board and member of its Finance Committee, felt that Mr. Greene should give due weight to his opinions. Given the temperaments of both men, it is not surprising that the course of their discussions was sometimes heated, but in the end both gentlemen allowed their basic interest in the enterprise priority over personal differences and devoted themselves to the various other problems which needed attention.[*]

On June 27, the CMB accepted the budget request of the Trustees as presented, authorized the College to settle exchange "at its option" by September 1, 1932, approved the transfer of the New York office of the PUMC to the CMB as of July 1, 1932, and in general appeared favorably impressed by Mr. Greene's reports on the situation in Peking. At Mr. Greene's suggestion a leave of absence was approved for Miss Eggleston to visit Peking in the autumn of 1932. On July 1, Mr. Greene heard from Peking that in accordance with the CMB authorization to settle exchange on the silver portion of the budget this had been done at the rate of 4.80

---

[*] One useful step taken at this time was a revision of the CMB By-laws more clearly defining the responsibilities of the Director and the Secretary in terms which neither Mr. Rockefeller nor Mr. Greene took exception to.

to 1, reducing by US$32,073 the amount needed to cover the budget which had been reckoned conservatively at 4.30 to 1.

One feature of the closing out of the PUMC New York office was the transfer of the Treasurer's office to Peking and the elimination of the post of Comptroller of the College by combining the duties of that post with those of the Treasurer. Miss Eggleston at this time succeeded Mr. Rockefeller, 3rd, as Secretary of the CMB, performing "such services as have hitherto been discharged in New York by the Secretary of the Board of Trustees of the PUMC." A local Secretary of the Trustees, Miss Mary E. Ferguson, Registrar of the College since 1928, was then elected in Peking.

Problems of Long–term Financing

When Mr. Greene returned to Peking in mid-August, relationships with the CMB and Rockefeller Foundation appeared smoother than for some time. It was a busy autumn with visits from Dr. Alan Gregg, who had succeeded Dr. Pearce as Director of the Division of Medical Education of The Rockefeller Foundation; Miss Margery Eggleston, Secretary of the CMB; Mr. S. M. Gunn, Vice President of the Foundation, and Dr. Victor G. Heiser, Associate Director of the International Health Division. Although the President, Mr. Max Mason, had been unable to make the visit which Mr. Greene had been urging upon him, the College was once again becoming a reality to responsible officers of the Foundation.

Dr. Gregg's visit was of special value. Like Dr. Pearce, his wide knowledge of medical education in the United States and Europe was coupled with wisdom and insight. Although he stayed in Peking less than a month, he left with an extraordinary understanding of the institution, its problems and needs, and its unique role in the developing, though confused, national health program of the Chinese government. Far-ranging discussions with the faculty, individually and in groups, as well as with Mr. Greene, came back constantly to the long-term financing of the College, something which was very much on their minds with the approach of June 30, 1933, the terminal date of the last of the five-year supplementary grants from The Rockefeller Foundation. There was complete agreement on the two major points: (1) the need for financial assurance for a long enough period (five to eight years) to make long-term plans and appointments, and (2) reduction of the uncertainties resulting from fluctuations in exchange. Together, Dr. Gregg and Mr. Greene drafted an informal proposal for the eight-year financing of the College and the CMB, which included the suggestion that instead of annual supplemental payments, the Foundation entrust to the PUMC Trustees a lump sum roughly equivalent to the total of the eight annual payments, leaving to that body the important task of its investment. They believed this would be sound preparation for the eventual turning over of the whole endowment to the Trustees as long envisioned by the Foundation. In the meantime, the risk of exchange fluctuations could be eliminated on about two-thirds of the silver budget by conservative investments in silver-bearing securities, as had been successfully done by the China Foundation, whose Executive Committee was almost identical with the members of the PUMC Trustees Executive Committee.

When Dr. Gregg left Peking in October 1932, he had agreed to keep Mr. Greene informed as to how and when the proposals for the new financing of the PUMC should be presented. On his return to New York, he found that the financial situation in the country in general and in New York specifically had deteriorated more seriously than he had realized while he had been away. He wrote Mr. Greene that "all institutions in this country are faced with reductions of varying degrees of severity." Examples were cuts at Boston City Hospital of 23%; Western Reserve with successive cuts of 15%, 13% and 11% and a further cut around 15% close at hand. The anticipated income of the Foundation during the year ahead would barely meet existing obligations without any new projects, with "greater pressure than ever before to keep out of the red." Early in February Dr. Gregg cabled Mr. Greene advising that the request for long-term financing go to The Rockefeller Foundation through the CMB, not directly from the Trustees, and indicated that this should be for five years, rather than the eight-year period discussed while he was in Peking. He advised that the estimates for developing the departments of public health and psychiatry be submitted as separate items rather than as a part of the overall planning for the future, and reported that under existing circumstances there was no possibility of effecting the transfer of capital to the PUMC Trustees which he and Mr. Greene had hoped for.

Dr. Gregg's cable reached Mr. Greene on February 1, 1933. On February 20, the PUMC Trustees held a Special Meeting at which they first considered the Operating Budget for 1933-34, and then took up the question of financing for the five-year period beginning July 1, 1933. The budget was approved in the sums of US$381,491 and Mex. 1,418,727 converted into gold at the rate of 4. 80 on which the exchange for the previous year had been settled, giving a total of US$677,059—a net decrease in the 1932-33 total of some US$200, but an actual increase of nearly Mex. 100,000. The risk of unfavorable exchange fluctuation remained but it was believed that this was covered by the CMB exchange reserve.

In discussing the question of financing for the next five years, Mr. Greene frankly stated that he found it difficult to look ahead on the basis of an annual decrease in income of US$10,000 a year from the CMB and The Rockefeller Foundation, and felt that if the budget could be held at its present level in the face of increasing demands for service it would be doing well. The Trustees were sympathetic with this point of view, and also agreed with the proposal that the five-year financing should include provision for extension of the activities of the institution to meet important needs in psychiatry and public health, and to cover opening of an additional ward in the hospital. Requests calling for total commitments of US$2,185,433 and Mex. 7,635,133 for the five years ending June 30, 1938, together with such provision as the CMB might find possible to safeguard the silver portion of the budget against possible impairment through appreciation of silver, were duly approved by the Trustees for transmission to the CMB.

These actions were promptly sent on to New York. Writing personally to Dr. Gregg, Mr. Greene pointed out that the supplementary subsidy the CMB would have to ask of the Foundation was only about 63% of that for the previous five-year period, and hoped this would create a favorable enough impression that the Foundation would not insist on an annual reduction. "If you must cut us down, do so, but pray cut as little as possible, every cut will hurt... even if the Foundation gives us all we ask, we shall have to apply ourselves strenuously to live within our income."

Mr. Greene's letter transmitting the proposal for five-year financing was received in New York on March 23. The inauguration of President Roosevelt on March 4 and the drastic measures he immediately set in motion to halt economic disaster, were very much in the forefront of everyone's thinking. It was in this context that the CMB met on April 10 to consider the proposal.

All of the members present—Mr. Vincent, Mr. Fosdick, Dr. Gregg, Mr. Rockefeller, 3rd, Miss Eggleston, Mr. Dashiell (Treasurer) and Mr. Debevoise (Counsel)—agreed that so substantial a request at this time would be likely to raise opposition and possibly jeopardize requests. There was a tendency in Foundation circles to think of the CMB as amply supplied with funds to meet any emergency needs of the College. After a full and frank discussion of the whole situation, there was general agreement that the time was not favorable to make any such request to The Rockefeller Foundation, that the CMB itself did not find the figures and supporting data submitted by Mr. Greene adequate for a convincing presentation, and that it would be better to defer application to the Foundation until answers to many questions were available. In the meantime, the CMB could meet the on-going needs of the College for the year 1933-34 in full by drawing on its own reserves to supplement the annual income on endowment.

The full amount for the budget for 1933-34. was thereupon appropriated exactly as requested. At the same time, a memorandum to The Rockefeller Foundation was adopted, explaining that a proposal for renewed long-term financing at this time would involve a "judgment upon the scope and scale of expenditure" at which the PUMC might be stabilized, a judgment the CMB was not yet ready to make, so that it seemed advisable to postpone any proposal to the Trustees of The Rockefeller Foundation for the time being.

This was followed by adoption of the text of a communication to be sent to the Chairman of the PUMC Trustees, Dr. Y. T. Tsur, from the Chairman of the CMB, Mr. Vincent, discussing at length the considerations which had determined CMB reaction to the five-year proposal— reduction in the income of the CMB and The Rockefeller Foundation with the impossibility of predicting the duration of "this period of financial uncertainty," and concern as to the potential obligations of the enlarging budget in silver against possibly less favorable exchange in the future. Mr. Vincent spoke of the drastic retrenchments, sometimes crippling or even destructive, being felt by educational institutions in the United States to meet the realities of reduced income. He ended with the flat statement that "The Trustees of the CMB feel that they have no choice in the matter of new proposals involving increased and increasing expenditures; they cannot give support to these proposals," and admonished the Trustees to regard the action of the CMB in covering the budget for 1933-34 "as a commitment within which the Trustees of the PUMC will exercise the degree of caution and economy rendered necessary... and as a confident expression of (CMB) faith in the administration of the PUMC, and in its disposition not only to maintain the function of the school on a 'standstill' basis but in addition to effect all possible economies within that appropriation."

Dr. Gregg had cabled Mr. Greene the essential facts right after the meeting, then sat down at once to write a long, personal letter of comment on the course of events leading up to these decisions. At one point, he said that he knew it would appear that the people in New York did not understand the necessities and opportunities of the PUMC, but pointed out that in Peking it was equally difficult to realize what had happened to institutions throughout the United States and the resulting repercussions upon the attitude of Foundation and CMB Trustees. He summed up their attitude by asking "What are the reasons for which the PUMC should grow, or increase salaries, when every institution in the United States and most that we know about abroad, are experiencing cuts superimposed on existent reductions and leading a year-to-year existence?"

Dr. Gregg knew that the PUMC and its expenditures could not accurately or fairly be compared with other medical schools, but should be examined on their merits. He believed the College was one of the major interests of The Rockefeller Foundation, and that an examination into the future made with equanimity, imagination and deliberate reflection would be of greater value ultimately to the institution than any five-year action by the Foundation limited by the considerations of the present moment.

The cabled information from Dr. Gregg arrived in time to be reported to the PUMC Trustees at their Annual Meeting on April 12. They took it calmly, expressed appreciation for the provisions that had been made for the coming year, and authorized the Treasurer to settle exchange as soon as possible for the silver requirements in the budget for 1933-34. Mr. Greene also showed less signs of distress in his subsequent letters than Dr. Gregg had feared.

Settlement of exchange for the coming year's requirements unfortunately ran into immediate difficulties. The American government having just renewed its gold export embargo, no Peking banks when approached by the Treasurer on April 20 were able to make an offer for this large contract, and in reaction to the embargo the bank counter rate fell within twenty-four hours from 4.32 to 4.02 to 1. Not only was the silver portion of the College budget for 1933-34 thus completely uncovered at that moment, but any eventual rate secured was likely to be a good deal less than 4.80, the rate on which the budget had been calculated. Watching the situation from New York the officers there cabled advice against settling any exchange contracts at that moment.

The summer of 1933 was a busy one at the College as well as in New York. Both sides were preparing for the intensive discussions in the fall when Mr. Greene would join the members and officers of the CMB and The Rockefeller Foundation in a detailed study of the basic questions on the long-term financing of the PUMC. The frank and free personal correspondence between Dr. Gregg and Mr. Greene was an important contribution toward developing an understanding on both sides of the differing points of view. A Committee was appointed by the Foundation to study the whole question—Mr. Fosdick, Dr. Angell of Yale, and Dr. David Edsall of Harvard—for which Dr. Gregg drew up a comprehensive Memorandum on the PUMC (July 14, 1933). After analyzing some of the problems of administration with responsibility divided between the CMB, the RF and the PUMC, stressing the importance of a thorough understanding of the purposes and methods of the institution, he submitted for discussion the suggestion "that the CMB be given by the Foundation a sum adequate for the CMB to be financially responsible" proposing specifically the addition of $8,000,000 to the existing capital of $12,000,000 held by the CMB, bringing the total to $20,000,000.

Dr. Gregg's memorandum ended with a section headed "Special Considerations in Connection with the PUMC", touching on distance from New York, delays of communication, cost of travel, freight, etc.; dangers and uncertainties of civil war, invasion, famine, and floods; fluctuations in exchange; the needs of foreign personnel for housing, furloughs, travel, education of their children, and protection in times of civil disturbance; the unavoidable combining of hospital maintenance with costs of education proper, making unfair a comparison of PUMC costs with medical schools not bearing this charge; the lack of adequate industrial and technical facilities so that the institution had to make its own provision for such things as power, water, gas and electricity, and nitrous oxide.

Mr. Greene could have made no clearer exposition, if indeed as convincing a presentation. The ground was prepared for the forthcoming discussion, and Mr. Greene himself wrote Dr. Gregg that he thought it entirely appropriate that the Foundation should consider the enterprise afresh "on its merits as a means of accomplishing important and interesting results... worth supporting on an efficient basis for another period, of from five to ten years." On October 4, he attended the first meeting of the Foundation committee in New York. Throughout October and November, there were numerous informal conferences, many of them with the financial officers of the Foundation and with responsible bankers on the question of possible investment in silver-bearing securities to meet the silver portion of the budget, a matter in which there developed considerable interest. Somewhere along the line, Mr. Rockefeller, 3rd, was named a committee of one to study this question. On November 22, he met informally with Mr. Fosdick, Dr. Edsall, President Mason, Dr. Gregg and Mr. Greene. According to a memorandum from Dr. Gregg to Mr. Vincent, Mr. Rockefeller presented his report "on the advisability and feasibility of transferring capital amounts into securities bearing interest in Chinese currency" and recommended delay for further study because of the divergence of opinion expressed by those whom he had consulted. Much of the discussion centered on a reduction in the PUMC budget for the coming year, possibly by $50,000. Mr. Greene's protests notwithstanding, there appeared to be general agreement that there was no reason why the PUMC should not accept reductions when these were being felt by institutions all over the United States and also by other Foundation programs. Both Dr. Gregg and Dr. Edsall pointed out, however, that the difference between the situation of the PUMC and other schools in this country made it desirable to avoid over-drastic cuts.

Mr. Fosdick then moved that a report be prepared for the Trustees of The Rockefeller Foundation in three parts: (1) an historical summary of the changing financial situation, reduced to the simplest possible terms and dimensions; (2) a recommendation that the contribution of the RF to the CMB for the expenses of the year 1934-35 be reduced by $50,000, (3) a recommendation that a transfer of US$5,000,000 be made by the RF to the CMB for investment into securities bearing interest in Chinese currency, this transfer to be made "if, as, and when," in the opinion of the Finance Committee of the Foundation, desirable securities were available, such a transfer to be considered as the first step in a program of eventual capitalization "in the neighborhood of $6,000,000 to $7,000,000." Dr. Gregg seconded Mr. Fosdick's motion and it was passed.

This appears to have been the last formal meeting of the Rockefeller Foundation Committee. On December 13, its report was presented at a meeting of The Rockefeller Foundation, following in general the three-pronged recommendations. It was agreed that the time was not favorable to the appropriation of capital funds in the amount indicated ($5,000,000) but, in addition to appropriating the funds requested by the CMB to enable it to cover a PUMC operating budget $50,000 less than the current year, the Foundation Trustees did authorize the Executive Committee to "appropriate sums not to exceed in total $1,000,000 to the China Medical Board, Inc., payments to be made in cash to cover purchases if, and as made, by the CMB, of securities bearing interest in Chinese currency for the capital funds of the CMB, Inc."

Mr. Greene had already left for Peking when these actions were taken by The Rockefeller Foundation and reported to the CMB, which at once referred to its Finance Committee consideration of the question of investment in silver-bearing securities of the $1,000,000 promised by The Rockefeller Foundation. Action was taken by the CMB notifying the PUMC Trustees that the budget for the year 1934-35 should be prepared in an amount at least US$50,000 less than that of the current year. Since Mr. Greene had taken part in the discussions of the Foundation Committee, this specified budget reduction would be no surprise to him, unpalatable though it was. The Board also approved an increase of its membership to seven, a step with which Mr. Greene was in full accord.

Among other matters discussed by Mr. Greene and dealt with at this meeting of the CMB was the matter of fire insurance on the PUMC buildings, and provision for the salary and expenses of an Assistant Director of the CMB to relieve Mr. Greene in Peking of some of his administrative load which the Board felt was unduly heavy. On both these matters, Mr. Greene differed with the officers of the CMB, basing that difference primarily on cost to the budget. He believed that self-insurance would protect the buildings against fire quite as well as commercial insurance, while at the same time relieving the tightening budget of more than $7,000 a year. The financial officers in New York insisted on the preferability of commercial insurance and prevailed. As for an Assistant

Director, he questioned the necessity for such an officer, suggesting instead a less highly-salaried assistant to the Controller. Again, the CMB preference was followed. On his return to Peking, he wrote Dr. Gregg his distress at the tendency of the CMB in matters where it had the deciding voice both to prevent possible economies and to add unnecessary expenditures to the budget, while at the same time pressing for other reductions in the budget which limited the effectiveness of College activities.

There being obviously nothing that he could do at this juncture, he accepted the situation and made the necessary adjustments with as good grace as possible. Looking back on his recent visit to New York, he wrote Mr. Vincent that he had found it "on the whole rather satisfactory, considering the financial position in the United States." He acknowledged that the impending cut of 5% in the budget was "trifling" compared with the reduction in most budgets in the United States, but reminded Mr. Vincent that when an American medical school eliminated some activity or reduced the efficiency of some service, it could usually refer students or patients to some other institution not too far away where such work was still available. The PUMC, on the other hand, had no other comparable institutions within reach, was still small and inadequate in terms of the role it was expected to play, and he hated to see its effectiveness lessened. In any case, he was glad he had been in New York and more warmly than his native restraint normally allowed, he said that at times he would be "quite discouraged without the sympathetic support which you and other friends in New York are giving to this enterprise."

1934 — Year of Crisis

Turning at once to the unpleasant but unavoidable task of drawing up the budget for 1934-35 with the cut of US$50,000 prescribed by the CMB, Mr. Greene called on heads of departments, divisions, and services to do their part in working out the necessary economies. When the resultant budget reached New York, however, there arose once again a sharp difference of interpretation between the CMB and Mr. Greene. Mr. Greene and the College Budget Committee had applied the $50,000 reduction against the total of $854,500 originally appropriated by the CMB for 1933-34. The officers and CMB members maintained that their understanding of agreements reached with Mr. Greene in New York (unfortunately not recorded in detail) was that the reduction would be applied against the *actual US dollar cost* of that budget to the CMB which favorable exchange rates had brought down to $838,083. The Board accordingly made a flat appropriation of $788,083 for operation of the PUMC for 1934-35, leaving it to the Trustees to make such adjustments between the gold and silver sides of the budget as the further reduction of some $16,000 might require. Cabled protests from Peking proving of no avail, there was nothing for the administrative officers of the College but once more to review the budget and make the necessary further cuts. Mr. Greene particularly resented this additional pressure since he felt that the original action of the CMB requiring the $50,000 reduction had been made not because CMB and RF income losses were that serious, but arbitrarily to keep the PUMC from considering itself *entitled* to continue in more favorable financial circumstances than institutions in the United States.

The day after receiving the cabled report of the CMB budget action, Mr. Greene received a personal letter from Dr. Gregg in the course of which he touched on a subject they had discussed together at various times in Peking and in New York—the sometimes anomalous situation of holding concurrent administrative responsibilities as Acting Director of the College and Director of the CMB, and the possible desirability of Mr. Greene's resigning the CMB directorship sooner or later. Dr. Gregg wrote: "The time has come for me to say to you what I told you I'd say if it seemed best, namely that I am quite sure you should resign from the CMB. You are in a relationship here now which you cannot rectify from China or wisely continue if it is not rectified. Your services are known and respected, but your advocacy of PUMC is feared because you are still in the Jury—i. e., the CMB. I am quite sure that your effectiveness for the future will be much facilitated by dropping out. I have no reason to think that advantage would be taken of your not being on the Board. Instead the resentment and fear which stand in the way of getting things done would be definitely less... I cannot say what the future will be but this next move is one to be taken before I can see any future at all... Do *not* become discouraged: to me the PUMC and CMB show more promise than they have for a year."

Mr. Greene's confidence in Dr. Gregg's judgment was so complete that he acted immediately by addressing a letter of resignation to Mr. Vincent, dated April 21, 1934, giving as his reason the desirability of simplifying "the somewhat complicated structure of our organization." This letter he sent to Dr. Gregg to present, expressing his hope that it might be held over to the November meeting of the CMB when he himself could be present to discuss the organizational implication of his resignation, but leaving Dr. Gregg full discretion to act as he thought best. Mr. Greene ended with an expression of the comfort he found in Dr. Gregg's "continued friendliness and confidence in my local administration, if not in my ability to conciliate those in the seats of power at home, as to which I confess I am a poor diplomatist."

Budget problems notwithstanding, the work of the College, School of Nursing, and Hospital was going on unabated. Graduate students came from all over the country for training tailored to the needs of each individual and the institution from which he had come. The clinics of the outpatient department were crowded to capacity. Hospital beds were in demand. Members of the faculty were frequently called to other places in China for special lectures, or for government service which seemed to assume priority over academic obligations. Staffing of the medical and nursing faculties was a never-ending problem. The death on March 15, 1934 of Dr. Davidson Black was a serious blow to the institution and a personal grief to Mr. Greene, creating a whole series of problems as to the needs of Mrs. Black and their children and the future of the paleontological research in which Dr. Black had played so significant a role.

Research in the laboratories of the Department of Anatomy first attracted widespread attention in 1926 when Dr. Black, on the basis of his study of a single fossil tooth excavated at Chou Kou Tien, west of Peking, identified a distinct genus of hominid. Subsequently this was confirmed with the finding of the first *Sinanthropus* skull at the same site—the world-famed "Peking Man". By this time the excavations and investigative program had come under the control of the Cenozoic Research Laboratory of the National Geological Survey of China of which Dr. Black was named Honorary Director. With warm support from both Dr. Houghton and Mr. Greene, laboratories in the PUMC were made available to the Cenozoic Research Laboratory, where Dr. Black and his Chinese colleagues, Dr. C. C. Young and Dr. W. C. Pei, with enthusiastic collaboration of Father Teilhard de Chardin, pursued the intensive studies which redounded so much to the credit of the PUMC. Beginning in 1926 The Rockefeller Foundation made substantial grants for this program, grants which were continued when, following Dr. Black's death, Dr. Franz Weidenreich, another distinguished anthropologist, came to the PUMC as Visiting Professor of Anatomy. Like Dr. Black he was appointed Honorary Director of the Cenozoic Research Laboratory continuing the cooperative study of the rich material being excavated at Chou Kou Tien where the original finds had been made.

By agreement all original papers coming out of the Cenozoic Research Laboratory were first read and published by the Geological Society, which also had the right of possession and disposition of all specimens excavated and collected under this program. It was under the terms of this agreement that in the late autumn of 1941, Dr. Wong Wen-hao, a trustee of the PUMC and a minister of state of the Nationalist Government in Chungking, sent word to Dr. Houghton in Peking on behalf of the Geological Survey of which he was then Director, instructing him to turn over to the commanding officer of the U.S. Marine detachment in Peking the original Sinanthropus skull and other material, for transportation to the United States with the effects of the departing Marines. Dr. Houghton was reluctant to do this, fearing loss or damage in transit of these irreplaceable specimens, but his instructions were explicit and he had no alternative. About December 6, 1941 the Controller accordingly personally delivered a locker trunk containing this material to Colonel W. W. Ashurst. It was put with the goods belonging to the Marines and taken to the port of Chingwantao, where the whole shipment was awaiting loading aboard ship when war broke out on December 7/8, 1941. Japanese anthropologists themselves did not credit the story that the *Sinanthropus* material had been sent away from Peking, and made exhaustive searches and inquiries at the PUMC and elsewhere in the city without success. No authentic information has ever been received as to its fate, but some who were in Peking at that time think it not unlikely that Japanese soldiers, breaking open Marine effects at Chingwantao in search of arms, ammunition, and other useful articles, may have come upon this locker trunk, found it full of old bones and skulls, and thrown the contents unceremoniously on the nearest dump heap or into the sea.

One action of the CMB at its meeting on the PUMC budget which had pleased Mr. Greene was the election of Dr. Houghton as a Trustee to succeed Dr. Paul Monroe, for he believed Dr. Houghton's understanding of the needs of the College would be helpful. Writing about Dr. Houghton's election, Dr. Gregg indicated that an important factor in bringing him on the Board was the possibility that he might be able to secure a year's leave of absence from the University of Chicago to undertake a study of the "whole concept of CMB-RF-PUMC relationships and organization," as a preliminary to "making such changes as will result in a better functioning than exists at present."

A letter from Mr. Vincent shortly after the meeting reported that the University of Chicago had been specifically asked to give Dr. Houghton a year's leave of absence. "If this is granted, Dr. Houghton will spend the summer months in the New York Office and then in September he will go to Peiping for a stay long enough to make possible a thorough understanding of the problems of the College. It is our hope that he will be able to work out with you and the Trustees the budget for 1935-36, and bring this back to New York in the late winter or early spring. " A second letter from Mr. Vincent said that the University of Chicago was reluctant to have Dr. Houghton away for so long a time, so that the plan might have to be postponed or modified, but he promised to keep Mr. Greene informed by letter or cable as the situation developed.

When Mr. Greene received Mr. Vincent's two letters, he realized how important it was that his own plans for going to New York in November and those for Dr. Houghton's visit to Peking should be synchronized, and at once cabled Mr. Vincent: "Your letters May 7 received. Unless Houghton can start immediately suggest he defer visit till I return November. Postponement my trip would gravely inconvenience institution." Mr. Vincent replied immediately: "Essential you be in Peiping three months from end August while Houghton there. Could you come immediately returning with Houghton" ? Mr. Greene lost no time in arranging matters, cabling on June 2: "Arriving Seattle 26th. Assuming opportunity consultation with Board and Foundation officers July. Wife arriving San Francisco 6th. Inform her." (Mrs. Greene, with their two children, had left in June expecting to spend the summer and fall in the United States, returning with her husband in the early winter).

Before he left Peking, Mr. Greene wrote Mr. Vincent about some of the points which would be coming up for discussion, and speaking especially of Dr. Houghton's election as "good news to me... it seems quite appropriate that he should visit us here. No doubt his reports on the actual conditions in the College will be most helpful to the Board. We can discuss the details of this visit when we meet in the United States, which I trust will be soon after you receive this letter."

Up to this point the record is clear that the general outlines of the plans agreed upon by all concerned in the China Medical Board, The Rockefeller Foundation, and the University of Chicago were that during the summer Dr. Houghton, while continuing his responsibilities in Chicago, would spend evenings and weekends studying reports, budgets, and financial statements sent to him from New York in preparation for the survey he would undertake in Peking in the autumn. In addition, he would come to New York the middle of June for a few days of conferences and again in August before his departure for Peking. On arrival in New York, Mr. Greene would participate in these conferences, returning to Peking with Dr. Houghton. Dr. Houghton was due back at the University of Chicago not later than January 1, 1935, President Hutchins having agreed with considerable reluctance to the persuasion of Mr. Vincent to give Dr. Houghton leave of absence for this purpose.

Mr. Greene landed in Vancouver on Tuesday, June 26, arriving in New York early the following week. On Wednesday, July 4, he met with Mr. Vincent—although this was a national holiday, Mr. Vincent was evidently clearing his calendar before an early departure for Europe for the summer. Mr. Vincent informed Mr. Greene that it would be necessary for Mr. Greene to resign not only the directorship of the CMB (which he had already done) but also the vice directorship of the PUMC, a post to which he had been appointed by the PUMC Trustees. According to Mr. Greene in a subsequent communication:

He was unwilling at first to give me any reason for this decision, but finally admitted that it was due to friction with the inner group of the CMB, namely, Mr. Fosdick, Mr. Rockefeller and himself. While maintaining that they appreciate what he called my good work for the College, he made it clear that my separation from the enterprise was necessary.

Anyone who has read the story up to this point must be fully aware of the existence of friction, and that tensions had been building up. No one was more aware of this than Mr. Greene himself, but he obviously had no conception of the intensity of personal antagonism to him that had developed among the officers and members of the CMB and the Foundation with whom he had so often and so vigorously contended for the support which he believed the College deserved. This had not arisen suddenly in response to some specific action of Mr. Greene's, but was rather a smoldering resentment kept alive by each successive altercation, ready to burst into flame at almost any moment.

That moment was determined by no less a person than Mr. Rockefeller, Jr. After his return in early June from a two-month Mediterranean cruise, he was briefed, among other things, on the continuing difficulties over the PUMC budget; on Dr. Houghton's election to the CMB and the plan for him to visit Peking in the autumn for a review of the College; and on Mr. Greene's expected arrival in New York about July 1. According to Mr. Fosdick, as he and Mr. Rockefeller, Jr., were riding uptown from the Foundation offices at 61 Broadway one June afternoon discussing the whole problem of the PUMC financing and administration, Mr. Rockefeller voiced his strong conviction that the time had come when Mr. Greene should be retired from the whole enterprise. Mr. Rockefeller had been intimately concerned with the establishment and support of the PUMC from the earliest beginnings in 1914; it was Rockefeller money which had made this possible through The Rockefeller Foundation of whose Board of Trustees he was still Chairman. It obviously never crossed his mind that there was anything unusual in his personal intervention, which even went so far as to name Dr. Houghton as his choice to succeed Mr. Greene.

Had Mr. Vincent, Mr. Fosdick, Mr. Rockefeller, 3rd, and others in the Foundation and CMB not already been so long irritated and disturbed by what they considered Mr. Greene's unreasonableness and inflexibility especially in budgetary economies which they felt inevitable and right, there might have been resistance to Mr. Rockefeller's dictum that as soon as possible after Mr. Greene's arrival in New York he should be instructed to resign not only as Director of the CMB but also from the post of Vice Director of the PUMC. As Chairman of the CMB Mr. Vincent agreed to handle this distressing task.

There is no question that Mr. Greene was taken completely by surprise and found Mr. Vincent's reluctant explanation that the action was due to "friction with the inner group of the CMB" vague and unsatisfactory. The very next day he asked Mr. Rockefeller, Jr., for an interview at which he pressed for a more explicit answer as to the reason for this drastic move. The session with Mr. Vincent had been a stormy one; that with Mr. Rockefeller seems to have been calm but uninformative beyond a statement by Mr. Rockefeller that he had "concurred in the decision."

Mr. Greene continued to seek for some more specific cause for his dismissal. On July 27, at what Mr. Fosdick described as a "long and painful luncheon," he pursued his search. According to Mr. Fosdick, "He was determined to get from me a statement of the exact reasons that led us to our conclusion in relation to him—and I was equally determined not to discuss details for I thought nothing would be gained by it."

What had made Mr. Rockefeller feel so strongly that he not only "concurred in the decision" but actually initiated it? Mr. Greene's insistence that the PUMC should enjoy a special status over and above universities in the United States receiving Rockefeller Foundation support, and his stubborn resistance to any cutting of the PUMC budget undoubtedly offended Mr. Rockefeller. He was later to state that things had reached a point where the CMB was obliged to insist that in acquitting itself of its responsibilities on matters of policy, its view and decisions should prevail over those of Mr. Greene, even though Mr. Greene might understandably feel that being on the field he was in a better position to reach wise decisions than was the Board. The situation which had developed was, in Mr. Rockefeller's opinion, "inevitable and could not have been avoided if there had never been any question of religious work in the College."

The mention in this context of the "question of religious work in the College" makes it desirable to review that aspect of the story, for it is hard to escape the conclusion that differences of opinion over the Department of Religious and Social Work were at least a conditioning factor in Mr. Rockefeller's decision to propose Mr. Greene's summary dismissal, rather than to lay out a more deliberate course of action which would lead to Mr. Greene's early resignation under less controversial circumstances.

The Christian Character of the Institution

From the first meeting of the China Medical Board in December 1914 which ended with Mr. Gates reading his paper, "Thoughts on Medical Missions and the Spirit of Jesus," there was a recurring emphasis on maintaining the Christian character of the institution. This was strongly stated in Mr. Rockefeller, Jr.'s letter of March 15, 1915, to the Mission Boards and was embodied in the Memorandum of Agreement with the

London Missionary Society dated June 2, 1915. Such phrases as "the most cordial and sympathetic cooperation" with the Mission Boards, and the hope of making "a distinctive contribution to missionary endeavor" appear frequently in official statements of the early years. At the Dedication Exercises seven years later, Mr. Rockefeller reiterated the same ideas: "In fullest sympathy with the missionary spirit and purpose, we are desirous of furthering it as completely as may be consistent with the maintenance of the highest scientific standards in the Medical School and the best service in the Hospital. We would ever show respect for the genuine spiritual aspiration, evidenced in service and sacrifice, of those who come within our doors, whatever their views—for after all, is it not a fact that the final test of true religion is the translation of that religion into the highest type of life" ?

The early implementation of these earnest commitments came through continuing the practice of the Union Medical College Hospital of employing "evangelists" who moved among the patients in the hospital wards and in the outpatient clinics, and the appointment of a "Religious Director" whose responsibilities were designed to include "social service work in connection with the Hospital of the College." There had been some expectation that the small budget for these activities might be met by the Mission Boards, but with the appointment on an interim basis for the year 1917-18 of Mr. Dwight C. Baker, the Trustees approved an item of Mex. 4, 050 in the College budget for the "Department of Religious Work," covering the salary of the director and an expense budget which included salaries of three evangelists. The mission boards were not asked to contribute to this or any subsequent budget.

Mr. Baker was succeeded in the summer of 1918 by the Rev. Philip A. Swartz, who served for four years. With the opening of the new hospital wards and clinics the need for a trained medical social worker was evident, and in February 1920, Miss Ida Pruitt who, in addition to her professional qualifications, had a fluent command of colloquial Chinese, was appointed to the staff of the Department of Religious and Social Work as "Social Service Worker." By the end of her first year of service, it was clear that administratively it was unsound for Miss Pruitt to be responsible to anyone other than the Superintendent of the Hospital, and on the strong recommendation of Dr. Pearce and Dr. Houghton she was transferred to the hospital staff. In the course of the next eighteen years, she broke the ground for medical social service in China and organized a highly efficient department in the PUMC where she not only trained her own staff but sent out workers who had an important influence on the development of social service throughout the country.

The scope of the program developed by Mr. Swartz for the Department, which continued to be called the Department of Religious and Social Work although the medical social service aspects had been moved to the hospital, ranged from work among the students, hospital evangelism, and the conduct of the College Sunday service to the physical education and recreational activities of the students.

At the week-long meeting of the Trustees in Peking in September 1921, it was agreed that on the expiration of Mr. Swartz's appointment in the summer of 1922, he should be succeeded by a "suitable Chinese." The choice soon settled on Dr. Y. Y. Tsu[*] as a man who could make an outstanding contribution to the College. It was the summer of 1924 before he was free to take up this appointment. In the meantime, a faculty committee headed by Dr. Houghton assumed responsibility for the Sunday morning services, kept an eye on the routine work of the staff of the department, and encouraged students in the organization of extra-curricular activities.

Once on the job, Dr. Tsu proved to be an admirable man for the post which he held for the next eight years. He was an excellent preacher in English as well as Chinese, and the College Sunday services attracted many persons, Chinese and Western, outside the PUMC community. The scope of the program did not broaden significantly beyond that laid out by Mr. Swartz, but Dr. Tsu's relations with students and staff, with schools and colleges in and around Peking, his standing among religious leaders in China, all combined to give the Department of Religious and Social Work a real place in the institution. It is not surprising, however, that whenever overall budgets began to be tight, there were some who questioned the presence in a medical school of such a department, whose budget by 1926-27 was comparable to those of minor departments in the medical school.

In 1927 as Dr. Houghton, Mr. Greene and the Trustees grew concerned over the possible effect on the institution of the educational policies of the

---

[*] An Episcopal clergyman then engaged in work among Chinese students in the United States under the auspices of the Y. M. C. A.

approaching Chinese Nationalists, Western missionaries and Chinese church workers were equally apprehensive over some of the anti-religious and anti-Christian attitudes of the new government. As early as August 1927, Dr. Tsu told Mr. Greene he was fearful that his department, as then constituted and named, might cause trouble for the institution when the Nationalists reached Peking. Mr. Greene advised Dr. Tsu that any suggestion of giving up the department would not be well received just then and even a change of name might cause anxiety to some of the Trustees. In any case, no immediate action seemed indicated at that time.

A visit to the College that autumn by Mr. F. H. Hawkins, the Trustee representing the London Missionary Society, was heartening to Dr. Tsu and also to the Trustees to whom Mr. Hawkins, on his return from Peking, reported "The work organized by Mr. Tsu and the members of his staff has helped the Trustees to carry out the promise made by the Rockefeller Foundation to the missionary societies when they handed over the College to the China Medical Board that its work should be continued as a distinct contribution to missionary endeavor." In April 1928, Dr. Tsu was reappointed for another four-year term.

As the various missionary boards proceeded with the formal actions that would put the College Board of Trustees on a self-perpetuating basis, suggestions were made that the original "appointing" boards be given "some guarantee" that the Christian character of the institution would be maintained. Mr. Greene was especially concerned that the new Board of Trustees, a majority of whom would be Chinese, should be a truly responsible and independent body unhampered by any "condition limiting the freedom of action," and he urged that no such commitment be required of them. In the end all the boards with appointing power, including The Rockefeller Foundation, took uniform action requesting the Regents of the University of the State of New York to amend the provisional charter of the College to make the Board of Trustees self-perpetuating, expressing in the preamble to the formal resolution their hope and expectation that this "would not interfere with the continuance of the Christian spirit and high purpose which had guided the management of the College since its organization." When the Trustees themselves, on April 11, 1928, approved the petition to the Regents they took a separate action expressing the same hope and expectation in the identical words used by the boards.

In terms of budget, the Department of Religious and Social Work was no more important than any other minor department in the Medical College. In terms of its role as tangible evidence of good faith toward the mission boards of The Rockefeller Foundation, and more particularly of Mr. Rockefeller, Jr., however, it was of major significance and unfortunately became a recurrent cause of friction between the officers in New York and Mr. Greene.

The first acute instance of this was in the autumn of 1928 when Dr. Tsu, who had just returned from leave of absence abroad, told Mr. Greene that he was unhappy over what he felt to be indifference and sometimes opposition to his program on the part of members of the faculty, and that he was thinking of leaving the College even though his appointment had more than three years to run. Mr. Greene was an admirer of Dr. Tsu, whom he described as "the best preacher in Peking... an ideal man for the position which he now holds" and although he himself had doubts as to the wisdom of maintaining such a department permanently, he hoped Dr. Tsu would change his mind and stay. In the meantime, however, it seemed to him wise to send a detailed report to the New York office by way of background in case it would be necessary to cable Dr. Tsu's actual resignation.

Mr. Vincent was greatly disturbed by this report when it reached New York, commenting to Dr. Pearce that to have Dr. Tsu resign under what might be regarded as pressure from other members of the staff "just as the new self-perpetuating regime goes into effect" would have a most unfortunate impact on the China Medical Board and the Rockefeller Foundation. He hastily sent off a cable to Mr. Greene expressing his distress, saying that Dr. Tsu's early resignation would be unfortunate and that the status quo should be preserved at least for the coming year, pending full consideration on Mr. Greene's visit to New York. In a covering letter, Mr. Vincent spelled out the basic considerations underlying the whole situation:

If you fix in mind (a) Mr. J. D. Rockefeller, Jr's letter which the missionary people regard as a charter, and (b) the resolution which was passed by the PUMC Trustees in connection with the change from the old to the new form of trusteeship, I am sure you will realize what the effect will be if almost immediately after the new regime goes into effect it is reported that an extraordinarily able and devoted director of the Department of Religious and Social Work had resigned because of the indifference or even antagonism of some of his scientific colleagues... The situation is so delicate and full of dynamite that it must be dealt with most cautiously.

By the time Mr. Vincent's cable reached Peking, Dr. Tsu had come to the conclusion that the situation was a good deal better than he had anticipated before his return, so that Mr. Greene was able to cable in reply to Mr. Vincent that Dr. Tsu was "happy and not contemplating resignation." Mr. Vincent by cable and letter expressed warm appreciation to Mr. Greene for having dealt with this problem "so promptly and effectively."

There the matter might have rested but for Mr. Greene's continued fear that the concern in New York over the Department of Religious and Social Work would impinge on the independence of the new Board of Trustees, a point on which he was highly sensitive. It was his view that if this Department were eliminated from the College budget, the funds previously designated for its support would be available for use elsewhere. Not so, replied Mr. Vincent. "This type of activity is so different from anything else the institution is doing that the CMB Trustees might take the view that with the dropping of the function the funds would also be discontinued." The irritating issue was still there.

It was raised again a few weeks later, this time by a special committee composed of two of the senior Chinese members of the faculty, Dr. C. E. Lim and Dr. Wu Hsien, who had been appointed to assist the Administrative Council in preparing the budget for 1929-30, with particular reference to possible economies in parts of the budget other than the salaries of the teaching staff. Their report listed among other suggestions the "elimination of unnecessary activities," one of which was the Department of Religious and Social Work whose work they commended but did not consider "a legitimate charge to the College budget." In passing this report on to the Committee of Professors, Mr. Greene pointed out that no radical change could be made during the existing appointment of Dr. Tsu, but that this was "a matter which can be dealt with on its merits in three years" when "some such change as is proposed will probably be desirable." No action was proposed or taken, but a copy of the report went to the New York office for information where Mr. Vincent undoubtedly saw it. In any event, the budget for 1929-30 showed no decrease for the Department of Religious and Social Work except for the elimination of the two evangelists, proposed by Dr. Tsu and agreed to by Mr. Greene.

When Mr. Greene was in New York in the spring of 1929, the chief order of business was the Annual Meeting of the College Trustees at which the actual revamping of the membership took place as described earlier, but there was also ample opportunity for discussion on many subjects of interest both to Peking and to New York. Mr. Vincent showed an understanding of the question of the appropriateness of "religious and social work" on the budget of a scientific educational institution, and suggested that some way might be found of providing the department's budget from outside sources, as in the case of the University of Chicago which had an independent endowment for its chapel. All were agreed, however, that no action should be taken during the term of Dr. Tsu's appointment.

Following the retirement from the Board of Trustees of the representatives of the mission boards, Mr. Rockefeller, Jr. was anxious to reassure those boards that he and The Rockefeller Foundation would do everything in their power to carry out in good faith the original understandings as expressed to them in his own letter of March 15, 1915, and subsequent statements. Accordingly, on June 20, 1929, he wrote to each of the boards and individuals concerned, pointing out that "although political conditions in China have hastened this change, it is after all only a step in the direction toward which we have had our faces set from the beginning. That the new board will carry on the traditions, scientific and spiritual, which were set up at the founding of the College and have been maintained ever since, is to be expected." He then once again made his personal commitment:

How deeply interested I have been from the outset in the spiritual possibilities of this institution, as well as its scientific possibilities, you well know. I need not assure you that I shall be no less alert in the future than in the past to do what lies within my power to preserve and perpetuate the fine Christian spirit upon which this enterprise was built.

A copy of this letter went to Mr. Greene who, thinking it a draft for his comment, advised against its being sent or of bringing the question of the Department of Religious and Social Work before the Advisory Committee for discussion as had been suggested. It was his opinion that the Trustees should be "quite free to maintain or discontinue this department as they see fit." An extensive correspondence ensued in which Mr. Greene, Mr. Vincent and Dr. Pearce took part, their letters crossing frequently en route so that the writers, with the best will in the world, never quite caught up with each other.

In one of these letters, Dr. Pearce agreed with Mr. Greene's position "that no officer of the Rockefeller Foundation should interfere with affairs of PUMC, or make demands or attempt to dictate policy," but went on to point out that "Mr. Rockefeller's position as an individual may logically be conceived as somewhat different in view of that celebrated letter that he wrote personally and not as an officer or member of any Rockefeller board. If he should be accused of going back on his personal word, he, and not the Board, would have to make good. This is the problem that bothers me, and not the points you discuss."

In the course of this exchange, it became evident that Mr. Rockefeller's present personal concern had arisen in part from letters addressed directly to him by several of the former mission board appointees on the old Board of Trustees. Mr. Vincent suggested that it would be sufficient to say in reply "that the new Trustees have raised no question about the Department of Religious and Social Work, that the present director is under contract for more than two years, that you have confidence that the new Trustees will seek to perpetuate the best traditions of the institution." This Mr. Rockefeller proceeded to do. The situation was quiet for the moment.

But not for long. One of the former trustees had a close friendship of long standing with a member of the PUMC faculty, who was in the habit of writing to him personally on various matters, particularly about faculty and administrative attitudes toward the Department of Religious and Social Work. This former trustee wrote in turn to Mr. Rockefeller. Mr. Vincent had retired from the Presidency of The Rockefeller Foundation in 1929. Dr. Pearce had recently died. Mr. Rockefeller turned to the staff of the New York office for information and comment and delayed replying to his correspondent for some months. By that time Mr. Vincent had returned to membership on the CMB to fill the vacancy left by Dr. Pearce's death, and Mr. Rockefeller could seek his counsel. The eventual reply was completely noncommittal, pending Mr. Vincent's return from a visit to Peking which he was planning in the near future on a leisurely trip around the world.

Writing to Mr. Greene before leaving New York, Mr. Vincent said that one thing he was especially anxious to discuss with him "fully and frankly," was the question of the Department of Religious and Social Work. "There are aspects and implications which, as you already know, give me some concern. From what you wrote me last, I assume that the *status quo* will not be changed without full notice. By that I mean that if the present incumbent were to raise the question of his future relationship, no decision would be reached before we have a chance to confer in Peking. I regard this as so important that I am writing this letter to make sure that you will not permit this matter to be considered, if possible, or in any event be settled adversely, before we meet. Forgive what you will doubtless regard as a quite superfluous precaution." Mr. Greene's reply assured him that there was no reason to expect any question to be raised prior to Mr. Vincent's arrival, but went on to say "I am myself much disturbed by the way in which the supposed autonomy of the College is apparently to be limited in respect to this matter. If pressure is brought to bear on the College by the Advisory Committee with some of its members in such influential position, it would be something to which I can hardly be reconciled."

Mr. Vincent's handwritten reply said, "Your paragraphs about the autonomy of the College disturb me also. I am not going to Peking on an official visit... I wanted to talk over with you in a perfectly informal, personal way a problem which seems to be difficult and important. I had hoped that we might come to see things in much the same way. I was anxious to make sure that the *status quo* would not change before my arrival. If, however, you feel that my visit would be misinterpreted or prove embarrassing don't hesitate to cable me to that effect... I am sure you will be quite frank with me." Fortunately Mr. Greene saw no reason for sending such a cable. Mr. Vincent's three-week visit did much to improve his relationships with Mr. Greene and with the Trustees for whom he developed a healthy respect. Their discussions on the Department of Religious and Social Work, together with Mr. Vincent's firsthand observation of the situation, resulted in a report to Mr. Rockefeller in the course of which he wrote that "the attitude of the Chinese Trustees turns out to be quite unexpectedly friendly to the idea of the Department. The Chairman, Dr. Tsur, made this most clear to me, so there need be no fear of antagonism from that source... On the whole, in spite of the probable loss of Dr. Tsu, the situation here is much more encouraging than it has been represented. I am confident that the present

Trustees will make every effort to support the Department as an agency for cultivating the right spirit and maintaining ideals in the College."

Dr. Tsu served out the full term of his appointment and his departure on June 30, 1932, was regretted by many, including Mr. Greene who would have been happy to see him stay on in Peking in some external relationship to the College. Unfortunately the time was not ripe for such an arrangement.

The budget for 1932-33 carried the same provisions for salaries and expenses as that for 1931-32, but no suitable replacement for Dr. Tsu having been found by the opening of the school year in the autumn, responsibility for supervising the work of the department devolved as it had more than once before on a committee of interested staff members with Dr. Maxwell as Chairman. Speakers were found for the Sunday services, student organizations and extra-curricular activities were encouraged, and the College community as a whole was not acutely conscious of the vacant secretaryship. Things having moved with reasonable satisfaction for a year without a full-time secretary, it seemed justifiable to Mr. Greene and the Budget Committee in making up the 1933-34 budget to provide only a part-time salary for the department head, in the belief that it might be easier to find an acceptable preacher to carry on the Sunday services than someone full-time who might not find sufficient outlet for his energies in an institution whose staff and students were immersed in their professional studies. The balance of the full-time salary was thereby released for professional departments which were feeling the pinch of economic pressures from New York.

Interestingly enough the PUMC Trustees themselves, when considering the budget proposals for 1933-34, brought into their discussions the future of the Department of Religious and Social Work although this was not on the formal docket for the meeting. A majority of the Chinese Trustees were in favor of maintaining the department on a full-time basis— both for the value of its service to the College and also because it seemed discourteous to oppose something so much desired by Mr. Rockefeller and his associates. Although reluctant to restore the full salary, Mr. Greene wrote to New York that he had "no recourse but to proceed in the manner favored by the majority of the active Trustees."

The availability just at that time of an American YMCA secretary who was well known to most of the Trustees as an excellent preacher and student worker was a fortunate circumstance. Mr. Egbert M. Hayes was very soon thereafter appointed Secretary of the Department of Religious and Social Work for two years beginning July 1, 1933. The additional funds to cover the full-time appointment were transferred from the budget of the department of pathology, which Mr. Greene felt was "robbing a scientific department," but under the circumstances there was nothing else to be done.

When Mr. Rockefeller Jr. learned of Mr. Hayes' appointment he wrote Mr. Greene expressing his "personal appreciation" of the happy conclusion to which you have brought this matter.

You will, of course, understand the peculiar satisfaction I take in what has been done in view of the fact that the original agreement with the missionary societies was based in no small degree upon my personal assurances as to the purpose and attitude of the Foundation toward the continuation of the religious spirit of the college as set forth in my letter of March 15, 1915, written as President of The Rockefeller Foundation. I realize that radical changes in thought along religious lines have taken place since the founding of the PUMC and that there is growing up a new school of thought as to how the fundamental and eternal principles underlying Christianity can best be promoted in the world and Christian character developed. On the other hand, so long as the PUMC stands, there can never be a question as to the duty of all those currently responsible for conducting the institution to carry out with sincerity and wholeheartedness the full spirit of the understanding with the missionary societies upon which it was founded.

After speaking of his gratification at the attitude of the new Board of Trustees, he spoke of the inevitability of the eventual replacement of the early missionary members of the faculty by others "who have not had that particular background and experience. That, however, must not be allowed to affect in any way the faculty's cordial and wholehearted attitude towards the carrying out of the understanding with the missionary societies which is as binding upon them and their successors as it was on their predecessors."

He then turned to Mr. Greene himself saying "how fully" he realized the difficulty of his position.

On the one hand not only are you fully cognizant of the assurances given the missionary societies, but you were a party thereto as one of the leading representatives of The Rockefeller Foundation and the China Medical Board when the pact was made. While on the other hand, you are now the representative of the Foundation and the China Medical Board in seeing to it that these assurances are lived up to fully although the Board of Trustees and the faculty have been in the meantime almost completely changed. If, however, both these bodies and their successors have laid before them from time to time by you, as occasion may require, the substance of the understanding above referred to, they cannot fall in line under your leadership in carrying it out as a matter of honor, even if not as a matter of conviction. And if at any time in the future a letter from me as Chairman of the Foundation to you or to the Trustees or faculty, calling to mind the basis of our agreement with the missionary societies and the obligation which we and our successors will always be under to carry it out, would be helpful to you, you have only to ask me to write such a letter...

This letter reached Peking after Mr. Greene had left for New York for budget discussions, and was forwarded to him there. While in New York in November 1933, he lunched with Mr. Rockefeller, one of the chief subjects of discussion being of course the contents of that letter. A few days later Mr. Rockefeller wrote Mr. Greene suggesting that perhaps it might be well for him to give a copy to the Chairman of the Board of Trustees, Dr. Y. T. Tsur, with such editing as Mr. Greene might feel desirable. Mr. Greene replied that he thought it would be better for Mr. Rockefeller to write directly to Dr. Tsur, using his letter to Mr. Greene as a basis, which Mr. Rockefeller did. Shortly thereafter Mr. Greene left for Peking feeling that his personal relationships with his colleagues in New York were satisfactorily smooth.

In January 1934, just after Mr. Greene's return, the College had a visit from Dr. Thomas Cochrane who was traveling around the world as senior Director of the World Dominion Movement and President of the Movement for World Evangelism. As Principal of the old Union Medical College and representative of the London Missionary Society, he had played an important part in the original negotiations which resulted in the College being taken over by The Rockefeller Foundation, and had continued to represent the London Missionary Society on the PUMC Board of Trustees until the reorganization in 1939 when, with other missionary trustees, he made way for the election of the new Chinese Trustees. Not having been in Peking since the Dedication Exercises in 1921, he naturally spent a good deal of time at the College and Hospital, understandably paying special attention to the Department of Religious and Social Work and Mr. Hayes. On Sunday, January 21, he preached at the morning service in the Auditorium. Mr. Greene wrote Miss Eggleston about this

104

visit: "I do not know what impression he has formed, but I gather he is fairly content."

Mr. Greene was evidently mistaken, for on March 26, when Dr. Cochrane was in New York on his way back to England, he wrote to Mr. Rockefeller, Jr. expressing great concern over the situation at the PUMC as it appeared to him. He felt that the staff was not being selected with due care "in relation to the idealistic aims of the College," and that the "religious director" should have "much more sympathetic cooperation and a better atmosphere than exists at present." He recalled how much he himself had been "comforted and cheered" by Mr. Rockefeller's attitude and assurances at the time of the original negotiations with the London Missionary Society and the other mission boards which had resulted in the establishment by The Rockefeller Foundation of the PUMC. The letter ended with an offer "gladly to go into this matter more fully" before his departure for England on April 3.

Only a sense of duty could have constrained me to undertake the unpleasant task of writing this letter. Men laid down their lives in founding this institution; they were medical missionaries, not merely missionaries of medicine.

The Institution is at the parting of the ways. It may become one of the greatest influences for good in all the Orient. But, I say it solemnly and advisedly, the Institution is on the downgrade in things which are most essential. China's greatest need today is not scientific medicine, but men of character. But the PUMC may meet both of these needs if present tendencies are checked and adequate attention given to a situation which I have indicated in moderate language.

Dr. Cochrane had struck a note certain to disturb Mr. Rockefeller who, however, had no time to go into the matter himself before sailing on a Mediterranean cruise on March 31. It was Mr. Rockefeller, 3rd, who at his father's request talked with Dr. Cochrane on April 2. He reported to Mr. Vincent that "the purpose of his visit to our office was to express doubts about the effectiveness of the Department of Religious and Social Work in view of the support which it is at present receiving. His letter outlines the situation as he sees it." Mr. Vincent's reply was characteristically wise and understanding:

I regret extremely that Dr. Cochrane feels as he does and I think I can understand in some measure why he is so deeply concerned. It is a difficult problem to combine an efficient training in modern medicine with evangelical piety.

He went on to say that he thought it would be well to leave it to Dr. Houghton, who would be going to Peking later in the year to make a study of the College for the CMB, to "deal with this difficulty."

This was just three months before Mr. Greene's fateful interview with Mr. Vincent. Mr. Greene's strained relationships with Mr. Vincent, Mr. Rockefeller, 3rd, and others whose support was so vital to the development of the PUMC, were of course significant, but it is hard to believe that without Dr. Cochrane's fortuitous intrusion on the scene just at that time, Mr. Rockefeller, Jr. would have acted as he did.

Mr. Rockefeller obviously believed that the results would be beneficial to the College, but he had failed to take into account the reaction of the PUMC Trustees when they learned that Mr. Greene, who was Vice Director of the College by virtue of their having appointed him, had been instructed by the Chairman of the China Medical Board, Inc., that he must present his resignation from that post. The structure of mutual respect and confidence between the Trustees in China and the RF and the CMB, that goal which had been shared on both sides of the Pacific and toward the attainment of which so many had striven over the years, had been rudely shaken.

The PUMC Trustees vs. the China Medical Board, Inc.

Technically Mr. Greene had not been dismissed; he had rather been instructed by the China Medical Board to resign from the vice directorship of the PUMC with certain stipulations. These included financial provisions for himself which would begin from the date of his leaving the administration, presumably December 1934; an undertaking to prevail on the Committee of Professors and the PUMC Trustees to appoint Dr. Houghton as his successor, and a pledge of secrecy on the whole situation until his return to Peking in September.

In the meantime, Dr. Houghton had been persuaded to give up his post at the University of Chicago to join the staff of the CMB on a full-time basis not yet fully spelled out. He would have preferred not to leave the University, but had agreed to the proposal on the insistence of Mr. Rockefeller, Jr., their long personal friendship making it difficult for him to refuse.

Both Mr. Greene and Dr. Houghton realized how easily word might leak out that Dr. Houghton was going to Peking on a permanent basis,

106

especially since his leaving Chicago would affect so many individuals in that institution's faculty and administration. They were right. By early August the news had reached New York via Cornell and New Haven, but without any reference to its bearing on Mr. Greene's status. Dr. Gregg and Mr. Vincent agreed with Mr. Greene, who thus far had meticulously lived up to the stipulation of silence, that he ought to write confidentially to Dr. Dieuaide, Acting Director during Mr. Greene's absence, and to Dr. J. Heng Liu, Director of the PUMC on extended leave of absence in Nanking as head of the National Health Administration. They would thus have facts with which to meet rumors that might arise.

Mr. Greene's letters were simple factual statements without any expression of his personal feelings. Copies were sent to Mr. Vincent in Europe who acknowledged them as "written in that spirit of consideration for the best interests of the College upon which I knew we could count." Probably no one of those involved in this whole unhappy situation was as conscious of its impact in human terms as Mr. Vincent, who had been called upon to carry it out. He ended on a poignant note: "I shall not see you before you sail. I send you my best wishes. Try to think of me as charitably as you can."

Before Mr. Greene left New York in mid-September, Dr. Houghton had made clear to the CMB as well as to Mr. Greene his personal distaste for the original proposal that the Committee of Professors and the Trustees be persuaded to name him to succeed Mr. Greene as Vice Director of the College. Not only was he unhappy at what had happened to his long-time friend and colleague, but he also had no desire to be imposed upon the College by fiat from New York. Dr. Houghton's expressed preference was an appointment as special representative or agent of the CMB with instructions to confer with the PUMC Trustees regarding relationships between the College and the Board, and to study at firsthand the affairs of the PUMC insofar as they might bear on those relationships. Dr. Gregg convinced Mr. Fosdick and Mr. Rockefeller, 3rd, that this was the wise course to follow, which is what was done. Mr. Greene was thus released from the obligation of persuading the Trustees and Professors to name Dr. Houghton as his successor.

On October 15, Mr. Greene arrived in Peking. He lost no time in fulfilling what he had been asked to do. His first step was to report to Dr. Y. T. Tsur, Chairman of the PUMC Trustees, submitting his resignation.

He then met with the Committee of Professors. In both instances there was amazed incredulity, with the immediate reaction that the resignation be withdrawn. The Committee of Professors unanimously expressed "satisfaction and confidence" in Mr. Greene's "policies and conduct of the institution," taking the unusual step of attesting this action by the signature of each member. This was reported directly to a group of four Trustees who were at the time conferring informally in an adjoining room. A week later there was a formal meeting of the Trustees' Executive Committee at which the general feeling of distress at Mr. Greene's resignation was again expressed. All agreed that resignation of the senior active administrative officer of the College was a matter of such great importance to the present and future welfare of the institution, that definitive action should be deferred for consideration by the full Board at a meeting to be called as soon as possible. In the meantime, the text of a cable to Mr. Vincent, Chairman of the CMB, was approved expressing "deep regret" at Mr. Greene's resignation. "In long association... we have found him conscientious, progressive, tactful, open-minded, impartial, efficient administrator. This estimate generally shared by Chinese intelligentsia and government circles. In all important matters he consults, secures approval Board's Executive Committee before acting. His administration successful in steadily raising institution's scientific standing. We feel retirement will be irreparable loss to the College." The cable ended with the statement that at a Special Meeting of the Trustees called for October 30, the Executive Committee would propose that Mr. Greene reconsider his decision, and the hope that this recommendation might "receive your endorsement and cooperation."

Mr. Vincent replied with a promptness which showed his realization of the seriousness of the situation, saying that the CMB members, scattered at the moment, would not be available to consider the message from the PUMC Trustees until after October 30. The proposed Special Meeting of the PUMC Trustees was accordingly put off until an official reply should be received from the CMB.

On November 2, there was a Special Meeting in New York of members and Trustees of the CMB, those present being: Mr. Vincent, Chairman; Mr. Fosdick, Dr. Gregg, Mr. Gumbel, and Miss Eggleston, Secretary. Mr. Rockefeller, 3rd, and Dr. Houghton were absent. There had been no formal meetings of the Board since June 14, 1934, when arrangements

Chairmen of China Medical Board

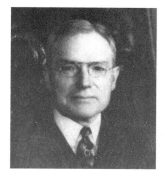 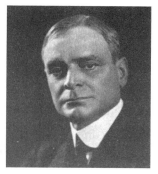

John D. Rockefeller, Jr.
1914-1916
President,
Rockefeller Foundation
1913-1917
Chairman, Rockefeller
Foundation Trustees
1917-1939

George E. Vincent
1917-1928, 1934-1936
President,
Rockefeller Foundation
1917-1929

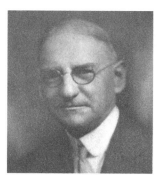

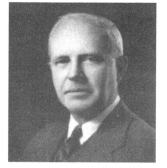

Philo W. Parker
1945-1956

Edwin C. Lobenstine
1936-1945

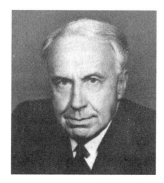

Raymond B. Fosdick
President,
Rockefeller Foundation
1936-1948

Superintendents of the Hospital

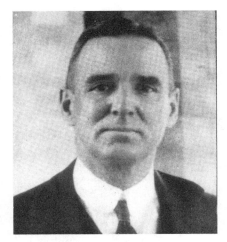

Dr. T. Dwight Sloan
1922-1925

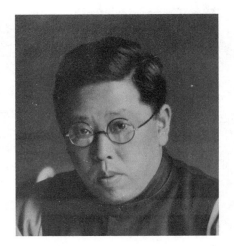

Dr. J. Heng Liu
1925-1934
Director 1929-1938

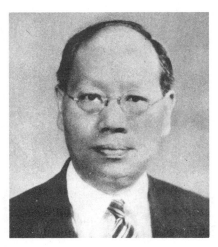

Dr. S. T. Wang
1934-1946

The "Peking Man"

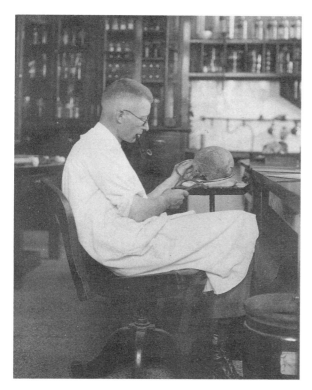

Dr. Davidson Black

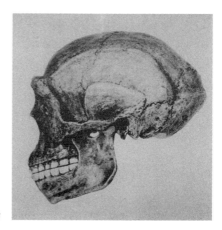

Sinanthropus Pekinensis

Deans of School of Nursing

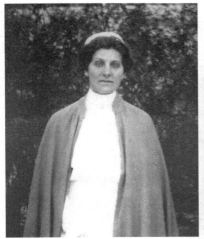

Anna D. Wolf
1919-1925

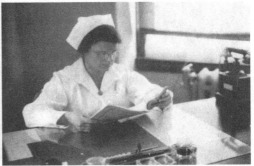

Ruth Ingram
1925-1929

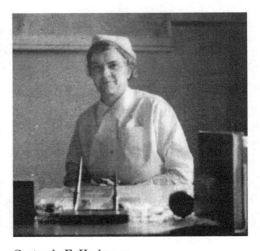

Gertrude E. Hodgman
1930-1940

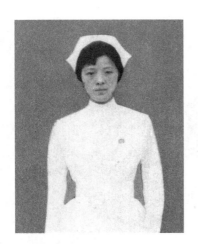

Vera Yu-chan Nieh
1940-

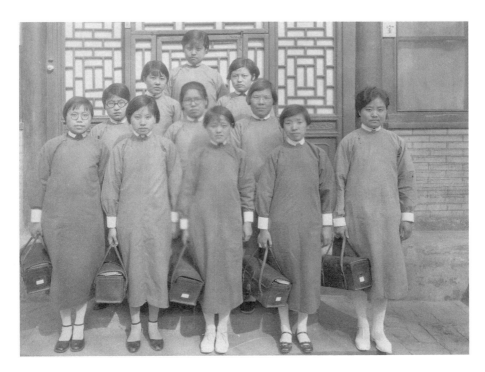

Public Health nurses setting out from the First Health Station.

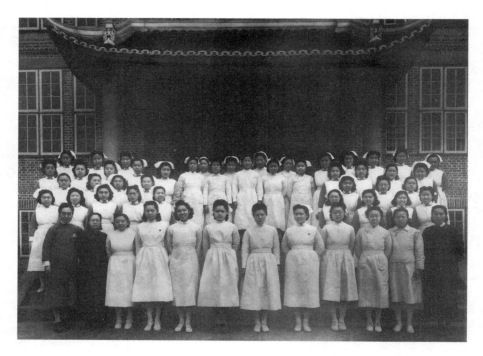

Staff and Students of the School of Nursing, Chengtu, Szechwan 1942-1946.

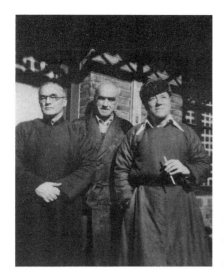

Dr. Houghton, Dr. J. Leighton Stuart and Mr. Trevor Bowen while under house arrest by the Japanese 1941-1945.

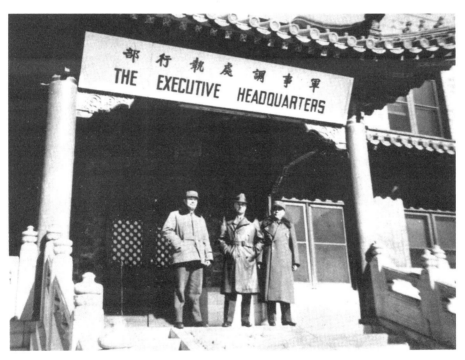

The PUMC houses General Marshall's Peace Commission, 1946-1947.

Rockefeller Foundation Commission—1946

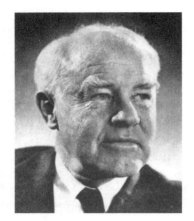

Dr. Alan Gregg, *Chairman*

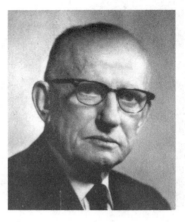

Dr. Harold H. Loucks

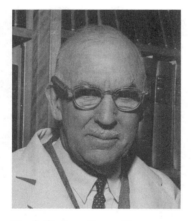

Dr. C. Sydney Burwell

Peking Union Medical College

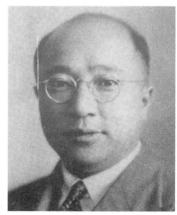

Dr. C. U. Lee
Director 1947-

had been approved for Dr. Houghton's six-month survey of the PUMC while on leave of absence from the University of Chicago, and where Mr. Greene's April 21 resignation as Director of the CMB had been presented. None of the momentous decisions of the summer of 1934 are recorded in the minutes of the Board. There is no record of the discussion on the communication from the PUMC Executive Committee at this early November meeting, but the approved text of the cabled reply to the Trustees shows keen awareness of the extreme delicacy of the situation in which the CMB found itself. It was drafted by Mr. Vincent, Mr. Fosdick and Dr. Gregg, three men of long experience in human relations and in the importance of the right words—words which would assuage, not exacerbate, the sense of outrage the PUMC Trustees were obviously feeling. The CMB reply, signed by Mr. Vincent as Chairman, started with an expression of appreciation of "the spirit of cooperation in the frank expressions of the judgment" of the PUMC Executive Committee. "The CMB recognizes that the actual administration of the PUMC is the responsibility of the Trustees of the PUMC." This was followed by a statement indicating the desirability of the two boards having functions that were "complementary rather than overlapping... maintaining distinct boards and officers... avoiding in particular the situation in the past whereby the acting director of the PUMC was also director of the CMB in China." After noting the further desirability of the CMB having a representative in China "who shall not be an officer of the PUMC" but "who shall serve as liaison officer between the boards and interpret the functions and needs of the PUMC to the CMB," it was reported that "the CMB Trustees have looked with favor on the proposal to name Dr. Houghton their representative at Peiping, and would be glad to learn from the PUMC Trustees if this appointment meets with their approval." The most important part of the message came in the next two significant statements: "The director or acting director of the PUMC will be responsible to the Trustees of the PUMC alone and the CMB recognizes the right and duty of the Trustees of the PUMC to determine appointments to their own board and to the staff of the College. The CMB is entirely willing to release Mr. Greene from his share in understandings reached last summer." The cable ended with one last word of reassurance: "The Trustees of the CMB view with satisfaction the development of the PUMC and share with its Trustees (in whom the responsibility for its efficient and useful functioning rests) the faith that it may become an increasingly important factor in the life of China."

It was not possible to get a quorum of the full Board of Trustees until November 19 but, in the meantime, the Executive Committee, acting on the basis of Mr. Vincent's cable, recommended that the full Board ask Mr. Greene to reconsider his decision to resign as Vice Director of the College. According to the Minutes of the Special Meeting on November 19, "the whole situation was considered from various points of view, emphasizing the paramount importance of the interests of the College in any action that might be taken." Following the discussion, the Trustees expressed their "high regard" for Mr. Greene's "integrity and devotion to the institution" and unanimously asked him to "reconsider his decision to resign from the position of Vice Director." The Chairman was authorized to cable the substance of this action to Mr. Vincent, expressing the hope that it might "receive the sympathetic understanding and support of the CMB Trustees." At the same time the Chairman cabled Dr. Houghton, cordially welcoming his appointment as CMB representative.

The cable to Mr. Vincent reached New York just as the CMB was holding its Adjourned Annual Meeting, after which the following reply was cabled to Dr. Tsur: "The Board appreciating your loyalty to the college recognize that the action you have taken was prompted only by the desire to serve the college's best interests and the board will, of course, continue to cooperate in every way."

When the adverse reactions to the CMB intervention with respect to Mr. Greene had begun to come in from the College Trustees and from many others in the educational, missionary and business communities in China, both Chinese and Western, Mr. Vincent quickly sensed the implications in relation not only to the future of the PUMC but also to the image of The Rockefeller Foundation. He felt that the one person who might be able to mollify the Trustees and help restore their confidence and cooperation was Mr. Fosdick, and he persuaded Mr. Rockefeller, Jr. to agree that Mr. Fosdick should go to Peking "to help straighten out the situation." At the CMB meeting on November 19, Mr. Fosdick was officially invited to visit China in the coming winter as a representative of the CMB, and a cable was sent to Dr. Tsur that Mr. Fosdick would be there in January to "confer on the interests of your board and ours." Promptly came the reply that Mr. Fosdick's visit would be "most welcome."

In the meantime Mr. Greene, in response to the Trustees' action of November 19 asking him to withdraw his resignation, requested time "to consider what action I should take." All the evidences of local support must have been heartwarming to him but these did not cloud his view of the other factors in the situation. He was anxious for comment and advice from friends in New York who had some personal knowledge of the situation. He also wanted to talk with Dr. Houghton on his arrival in Peking, for he was deeply concerned about the immediate administration of the College should he himself leave at the end of December as originally proposed. On the other hand, he did not want his continued presence to jeopardize still further the relationship between the College Trustees and the two New York boards and thus adversely affect the financial support of the institution.

By the time Dr. Houghton reached Peking on December 28, Mr. Greene's advisers in New York had told him that in their opinion his staying on as Acting Director "for the present" would not have unfavorable consequences for the College, although they questioned the advisability of a prolonged continuance. Dr. Houghton concurred in this advice and Mr. Greene accordingly withdrew his resignation, but in the personal expectation of submitting it again when this could be done without any undue disruption of orderly administration. Writing to Dr. Gregg about having withdrawn his resignation, he said he was sure that he should plan for leaving "but when"? The faculty would be again disturbed when the professors were called upon to nominate a successor, but "something must be done without too long delay if anything approximating academic calm is to be restored to the College."

Dr. Houghton stayed in Peking for three weeks as the guest of Mr. And Mrs. Greene. Not only did this give them easy opportunity to talk privately, but it was also visible evidence that their personal relationship was still friendly. During this time Dr. Houghton reacquainted himself with the College, its personnel, and with the Trustees. After conferences in Nanking with Dr. J. Heng Liu and others in the National Health Administration, he met Mr. Fosdick in Shanghai early in February. Together they visited Hong Kong, Canton and Nanking before going to Peking where they spent nearly a month, again as guests of the Greenes, until Mr. Fosdick's departure on March 16.

While in Peking, Mr. Fosdick conferred personally with all the available Trustees, establishing a rapport with them each individually. They found him ready for full and frank discussion of the whole situation. To direct questions as to whether the appointment of their officers did not rest with the Trustees, he answered that in the case of a new director or vice director selected by the Trustees of the College themselves, the CMB would never think of interfering, but that in the case of Mr. Greene the CMB had felt a responsibility because his connection with the College had come through the CMB. Out of these conferences came a growing understanding that the crisis of the previous year involved more than friction and clashes of personality. Basically it was the old question of relationships among the PUMC, the China Medical Board and The Rockefeller Foundation that was at issue.

Three days before Mr. Fosdick left Peking, the Trustees held their Annual Meeting. This he did not attend, emphasizing the fact that his mission had been to establish personal understanding with the members of the board rather than to participate in its formal business. At this meeting Mr. Greene once again submitted his resignation, having concluded as a result of his own conversations with Mr. Fosdick as well as with Trustees who had talked with the emissary from New York, that a satisfactory basis for future relationships between the PUMC and the CMB could "hardly be arrived at unless I were out of the way or unless the CMB, on the basis of Fosdick's report and discussion with the new (CMB) members, should change its mind about me."

Before Mr. Fosdick left Peking, he had an understanding with Dr. Tsur, Chairman of the Trustees, that he would report to the CMB the Trustees' wish to keep Mr. Greene, and would cable Dr. Tsur whether there was any change of heart among CMB members. If their opinion should be unchanged, the Trustees would accept Mr. Greene's resignation. Pending word of the reaction, the resignation was referred to the Executive Committee with power to act.

Late in April Mr. Fosdick cabled Dr. Tsur as he had promised, reporting no change in the general attitude of the CMB with regard to Mr. Greene. Mr. Greene at once told the Committee of Professors that he wished to resign as of June 30, and urged them to begin consideration of arrangements for the administration of the College beginning July 1. The professors, taking note that the broad future policies of the College would not be clear until the report then being drawn up by Dr. Houghton had been considered by the Trustees of the College, concluded that it would be difficult to make any arrangements for the administration other than a temporary one. They accordingly recommended that for the year 1935-36 the administration be vested in a Committee of three professors, the chairman to take the place of the acting director on all administrative committees of the College and Hospital, and to work in close cooperation with the Chairman of the Board of Trustees in all official correspondence. By ballot the professors nominated Dr. J. P. Maxwell, Dr. Robert K. S. Lim, and Dr. Wu Hsien for this committee.

On June 8, 1935, the Executive Committee of the Trustees "with deep reluctance" accepted Mr. Greene's resignation effective June 30, 1935, and appointed the Administrative Committee as proposed by the professors. On recommendation of Dr. Lim and Dr. Wu, the Trustees also appointed Dr. Maxwell Chairman of the committee with power to sign official papers as Acting Director.

On July 1, 1935 Mr. Greene turned over the administration of the College to the Administrative Committee. He was still a member of the Board of Trustees, having been re-elected for a three-year term at the same meeting on March 13, 1935, when he submitted his resignation as Vice Director for the second time. This was only one of the many ways in which the Trustees demonstrated their confidence in him. For the next three years Mr. Greene remained in official contact with the institution through the dockets and minutes of the Trustees, although he never attended any subsequent meeting of the board.

Administratively, as far as Trustee-CMB relations were concerned, the period between Mr. Fosdick's departure in mid-March and mid-December when Dr. Houghton presented to the CMB his report on the organization and program of the PUMC, was quiet. It was, however, a period in which the institution went through a most disturbing internal experience, potentially destructive of the exceptionally fine esprit de corps and excellent working relations that had grown up between the Chinese and Western members of the faculty.

It was a rude shock when in December 1934 grapevine rumors were confirmed by the overt action of several American staff members who, taking advantage of Mr. Greene's shaky status with the CMB, attempted to enlist Chinese colleagues in a conspiracy to oust the professor and head of a major department in a move to get control and reshape it to their own advantage. The Chinese loyally rejected these approaches and promptly reported them to Mr. Greene. For the next six months, although convinced that his own days were numbered, Mr. Greene was as much involved in this distressing situation as he was with his own difficulties. After various attempts to keep matters from coming to a crisis had failed, the three dissidents were dismissed on the unanimous recommendation of the Committee of Professors. The group then resorted to legal action before the extraterritorial U.S. Supreme Court for China, charging wrongful dismissal and demanding damages. On Saturday, June 29, just two days before Mr. Greene's resignation took effect, Judge Milton J. Helmick who had sat in extraordinary sessions in Peking for ten days in May, ruled that the dismissals were "in no sense wrongful... call for the imposition of no damages" and had been "for the good of the College," but that the men were entitled to the payment of salary and traveling expenses "which would follow any unexpected termination of appointment" (as indeed had originally been offered by Mr. Greene).

The next two weeks Mr. Greene spent working with the College lawyers on a suit for malpractice brought against the institution at the instigation of one of the dissidents. Not until this suit was dismissed by the judge without trial as completely unsubstantiated, did Mr. Greene join his family at the seaside resort of Peitaiho. A month later, the whole Greene family left for the United States.

For twenty-one years, beginning when he was thirty-two, Mr. Greene's life had been focused on the PUMC. As a member of the first China Medical Commission of the CMB he had participated in the recommendations which resulted in the establishment of the College; as Resident Director of the CMB he had been intimately involved in the building program and the many problems of administration and finance in the early years when the solid foundations were being laid; as Vice Director and Acting Director of the institution, his chief interest was in promoting the highest standards of performance possible through quality of personnel and adequate financial support. Now the College's future must rest in other hands than his. It was a sad moment for his friends and colleagues; it must have been a bitter moment for him, but a proud one too as he looked back over the years of the institution's growth and accomplishments.

In the meantime, Dr. Houghton had been trying to familiarize himself again with the institution in which he had once been so much at home. If Mr. Greene had been put in an uncomfortable situation by the China Medical Board's actions, the same was true of Dr. Houghton. He himself once wrote somewhat ruefully that "to the staff, generally speaking, the China Medical Board is a mysterious and hostile body of which I am the visible expression." He felt great personal sympathy for Mr. Greene, a fact which made his task of preparing a report of the Board in New York on the College's current condition not at all an easy one. Rather than moving around the various departments, asking questions of often resentful faculty members, he chose to keep himself very much in the background, spending a good deal of time in other parts of the country— Nanking, Shanghai, Canton—feeling out the reactions of responsible Chinese government officials, lay as well as medical; acquainting himself with other outside attitudes toward the PUMC, in the "foreign" communities as well as among the Chinese; assessing the political situation and its implications for the future of the College. When the Administrative Committee took over from Mr. Greene on July 1, Dr. Houghton was in Peitaiho where he spent the greater part of the summer working on his report, thus underlining the fact that the new administration had full responsibility and control.

At the Annual Meeting of the Trustees on March 13 which, like Mr. Fosdick, he did not attend, Dr. Houghton was elected a member of the Board. He had sat in on most of Mr. Fosdick's conversations with the Trustees, individually and collectively. At the last one of these with Dr. Tsur, Chairman of the Trustees, Mr. Fosdick suggested with the warm concurrence of Dr. Houghton, that in "the appraisal studies of the College which the China Medical Board had asked him to make" Dr. Houghton be assisted by a small committee of medical educators appointed by the Trustees. The Executive Committee also thought well of this suggestion and appointed a committee "to assist and advise" Dr. Houghton, naming Dr. J. Heng Liu, Dr. R. K. S. Lim, Dr. G. Canby Robinson, Visiting Professor of Medicine, and Dr. Charles N. Leach, Visiting Professor of Public Health as members.

Dr. Houghton returned to Peking in mid-September a few days before a Special Meeting of the Trustees on September 20, which had been called to deal formally with an application to the Regents of the University of the State of New York for replacement of the College's provisional charter by an absolute charter. He was due to leave on September 24 for New York to present his report to the CMB, and the Trustees were hoping that Dr. Houghton would show them the report and discuss his findings with them at that meeting. Dr. Houghton, however, felt that as his report was prepared at the request of the CMB, any formal discussion of it before it had been presented in New York would be not only premature but inappropriate. When he learned that the Chairman, Dr. Tsur, was disappointed at what seemed to be a bypassing of the Trustees, Dr. Houghton informed him that he would be glad to provide him with a copy of the report for his personal information. Dr. Tsur's response was that unless copies were available to all members of the Board, he preferred not to receive one. Wishing above all else to avoid offending the Trustees, Dr. Houghton had copies of the report hastily prepared and in the hands of the Trustees at the meeting. According to the Minutes, Dr. Houghton "made a brief statement summarizing the substance of the report which he had prepared for the China Medical Board, Inc." Discussion of its content was reserved until this had been considered by the CMB, and resulting comments returned to the PUMC Trustees.

In the meantime, the College and Hospital were carrying on normally under the direction of the new, albeit temporary, regime of the Administrative Committee. Entrance examinations produced the largest class yet accepted for admission to the Medical College—thirty, of whom five were women; the total undergraduate enrollment when the school year began on September 12 was 113, with an additional 72 graduate students, including 10 in the annual special intensive course in obstetrics and gynecology. The School of Nursing had 41 undergraduate students. Faculty who had been on furlough or abroad on fellowships returned to duty, while others left for similar opportunities. New appointees took up their responsibilities. The hospital wards had an average bed occupancy of 88.7%, the report of the hospital superintendent for 1935-36 mentioning the fact that during October and November "political unrest in North China somewhat disturbed the attendance in both public and private outpatient clinics and reduced the number of hospital patients. All services, however, were called upon to capacity during the balance of the year." The annual Bibliography of Publications from the various laboratories and departments for the year 1935-36 lists a total of 189 articles. In all significant respects, the institution was demonstrating its essential soundness.

The scene now shifts to New York. Dr. Houghton arrived there the first week in November but it was December 17 before a quorum was available to give formal consideration to his report on the Organization and Program of the College. In the 57-page report, Dr. Houghton voiced no harsh criticisms of existing practices nor did he recommend radical changes in program or direction. Even his discussion of the Department of Religious and Social Work summarized the basic elements of the situation in much the same terms as had Mr. Greene, including the statement that "one is brought inescapably to the conclusion that a different approach must somehow be made... Just how and when these changes should take place is a matter for thoughtful reflection."

Basically, what he had done was to pull together in one convenient document information which for the most part was in the regular reports and communications sent previously to the CMB from Peking. Dr. Gregg had once perceptively remarked that "The trouble is not that there is not enough information which can be specifically called for but that there is not enough understanding in New York of what the PUMC should have and can do." The fact of the matter was that Mr. Greene had become *persona non grata* so that reports from him lacked the confidence of the CMB. Dr. Houghton on the contrary had the Board's full confidence. His "State of the College" report was accordingly received "as a basis for consideration," with an expression of "appreciation of the extreme care, skill, and sympathy with which he had prepared his studies."

Appended to his report was a seventeen-page analysis of the Political and Military Situation in North China where the Japanese were increasingly aggressive. What bearing might this have on the future of the PUMC? He concluded that "other things being equal the work of the College is not likely to be greatly disturbed, even if a buffer state should be created out of the northern provinces... There seems to be no occasion at the present time for anxiety over these possibilities... political conditions in the Far East are in a highly fluid state, and... likely to be unstable and indeterminate for several years to come. No one can foresee what a few years—or even months—may bring to pass; so that until a critical change affecting the program of the College is clearly in view, no preparatory steps of a positive character need be taken. Negatively, however, the Board will need to be very cautious about the shifting of endowment funds to China, or in other ways exposing the Chinese Trustees to difficult and perplexing situations during this period of change and uncertainty."

Among the points raised by the College Trustees with Mr. Fosdick was their need for closer mutual understanding with the CMB and The Rockefeller Foundation on the fundamental basis of policy. This was reported by Mr. Fosdick and quickly followed up by a cordial letter to Dr. Tsur from Mr. Vincent, writing that "in accordance with your suggestion you will receive before long an official letter in which the relationships between The Rockefeller Foundation, China Medical Board, Inc., and the PUMC will be set forth in what I trust will prove to be a definite and satisfactory way." The letter ended with warm endorsement of Mr. Fosdick's invitation to Dr. Tsur to visit the United States at his convenience as the guest of the CMB and assurance of "a most hearty welcome here."

A few days later the promised statement of relationships was sent to Dr. Tsur. Mr. Vincent prefaced his five-page analysis with the hope that it might serve "to clarify a situation which perhaps has been somewhat confusing." He stressed the fact that the outline as drawn up represented "the situation as it exists in our minds at the present moment" with the possibility that "the facts and conclusions resulting from Dr. Houghton's study may somewhat qualify the comments herein contained." He dealt with the relationship to the College of: (1) The Rockefeller Foundation; (2) the China Medical Board, and (3) "the China Medical Board's representative." Mr. Vincent ended with the hope that his letter would make "reasonably clear the relations of the three boards," and the assurance of "the confidence we feel in the Trustees of the PUMC and in your headship."

Mr. Vincent's formulation of these relationships, based on his long and intimate involvement in each of these related boards, was the first step in the process of arriving at a definitive statement, acceptable to both the China Medical Board and the PUMC Trustees, in the drafting of which the Trustees in Peking took part. The next step was the appointment by the CMB, following the presentation by Dr. Houghton of his reports, of a Committee of Three—Dr. Alan Gregg, Dr. Alfred E. Cohn, and Dr. Houghton—to prepare "a general statement to be presented to the Trustees of the College concerning the principles and ideals by which this Board feels the development of the College should be guided, within recog-

118

nized limits of financial support." When Dr. Houghton sailed from San Francisco on February 8, 1936, he had in his hand the final text of a statement which had been intensively worked over by the committee and other members of the board, and had the official approval of the CMB.

This statement, which included a number of basic questions to be answered, was studied and discussed by the Trustees in the course of the next few months. The result was a succinct single-page document approved by the Trustees on September 26, 1936, for transmission to the CMB for consideration. The members of the CMB in their turn studied this version, accepted its substance, and returned to the Trustees a fresh two-page statement covering the same points, but somewhat expanded to make sure that each point was crystal clear. On March 27, 1937, the statement in this form was approved by the Trustees without question. The PUMC Trustees and the members of the CMB had finally achieved the specific definition of functions and relationships.

The Survey Commission

Before Dr. Houghton left New York he had been named Director of the China Medical Board. On March 1, 1936, he arrived in Peking to embark on the next phase of his commission from the CMB—establishment of clear limits of the degree of support which the College could expect from New York, and adjustment of program and personnel within those limits.

He found the groundwork already laid during his absence in connection with the preparation of the Operating Budget of the College for 1936-37 which was the responsibility of the financial officers in consultation with the Administrative Council. On February 18, 1936, when the budget was finally commended to the Trustees for adoption, the Administrative Council had also recommended that the Trustees appoint a commission "to formulate a statement of the policies and objectives of the College, to make an impartial and intensive survey and study of the institution and its financial requirements in the light of those policies and objectives, and to report its findings and recommendations to the Trustees." The recommendation went on to propose that Dr. Houghton be appointed chairman of the proposed commission which should be made up of the heads or acting heads of all academic departments, the Superintendent of the Hospital, the Dean of the School of Nursing and the Treasurer, with the Controller of the College serving as financial adviser to the Commission. These proposals were described as "recommendations of the Controller."

The Controller there referred to was Mr. Trevor Bowen who had been in Peking since March 4, 1935, under appointment by the CMB as financial adviser to Dr. Houghton. Previously he had served as Controller of the Institute of Social and Religious Research, a Rockefeller-supported organization in New York, which was disbanded in September 1934. There he had a record of holding the various projects undertaken by the Institute within their original budgets—an admirable qualification for the kind of fiscal control the CMB was seeking for the PUMC.

Not long after his arrival in Peking, Dr. Houghton and Mr. Bradfield, Treasurer of the College, agreed that Mr. Bowen could best familiarize himself with the College business administration if he were closely associated with actual operation of the financial machinery. On their recommendation he was appointed Controller of the College concurrently with his CMB responsibilities as financial adviser to Dr. Houghton in the preparation of his report. This gave Mr. Bradfield welcome assistance with his heavy administrative load without adding to the budget, since Mr. Bowen would remain on CMB salary.

As Controller, Mr. Bowen attended the meetings of the Administrative Council and participated in screening departmental budget requests for 1936-37. He knew that an important phase of Dr. Houghton's commission from the CMB was to see this budget substantially reduced from that for 1935-36, a point which he emphasized to the Administrative Council. In the end, the net decrease amounted to only US$6,598 but this was accepted by the CMB as a step in the right direction.

Mr. Bowen's recommendations for the appointment of a commission to assist Dr. Houghton in making his survey of the College reflected his understanding of Dr. Houghton's thinking. When, therefore, they were presented to the Trustees at the Annual Meeting on March 11, 1936, only ten days after Dr. Houghton's return to Peking, he readily endorsed them and they were duly approved by the Trustees.

No time was lost in setting the survey in motion. On March 16, 1936, at the call of Dr. Maxwell, Chairman of the Administrative Committee and ex-officio Acting Director of the College, all those designated by the Trustees to serve on the Survey Commission as recommended by the Administrative Council, met for its formal constitution under the chairmanship of Dr. Houghton. The only absentee was the Treasurer, Mr.

Bradfield, who had left a few days earlier on a long-delayed furlough and was absent throughout the survey.

At the outset, Dr. Houghton summarized the preliminary objectives of the survey: (1) entire freedom of action with respect to methods of examination, selection and preparation of data, and the nature of the conclusions and recommendations, "subject only to the restriction of the general objectives for which the institution was established, as set forth in 1921 and reaffirmed in 1936;" and (2) without any given figure as to the limit of funds available for the operation of the College, to bear in mind the desirability of "designing for economy as an achievement admirable in itself, and to note certain natural limitations of program."

A week later the Commission adopted recommendations for four subcommittees on (1) Educational Policy, (2) Cost of Operation, (3) Constitution and By-Laws, and (4) Religious and Social Work. Between April 13 and September 1, there were no meetings of the Commission as a whole, but those months saw the senior staff members appointed to the subcommittees spending many hours, in addition to their teaching, administrative and clinical responsibilities, in serious and intensive study of the terms of reference under which they were to formulate findings and recommendations to the Trustees.

In early June, Dr. Houghton was obliged to furnish the Commission and the Trustees information received from Mr. Fosdick, who was due to assume the presidency of The Rockefeller Foundation on July 1, that the income of the CMB had shrunk to approximately one-half that anticipated at the time of its incorporation, and that the income of the Foundation, from which the supplementary grants to cover the College budget had come, had suffered a corresponding decrease. This meant that reduced costs must now take precedence over quality of program, and that the efforts of the Commission must be directed toward finding "the lowest practicable level" at which the institution might operate.

While the subcommittees painfully adjusted their sights to this unanticipated situation, Dr. Houghton wrote to Mr. Fosdick analyzing the factors involved "in looking forward to the steps you propose... for in my judgment they have an important bearing on the Foundation's program in the Orient, no matter what solution of the immediate difficulties may be elected by the Board." In words often reminiscent of many of Mr. Greene's earlier analyses, Dr. Houghton's objectivity began to be tinged with partisanship for the College: "The College does not stand by itself. In the fifteen years of its recent history it has acquired a special setting and significant relationships that cannot be ignored in the making of a program for its continuance... As far as medical science and education are concerned, this is the outstanding institution in Asia... Only last week the Chinese Government made an informal approach... that through a small non-political intermediary body, this College should take charge of teacher training in medicine and nursing for the country as a whole... Whatever official name be applied to the College, it is known all over the world as a Rockefeller unit; this may be regrettable, but it is noteworthy." He pointed out that the registration of the College by the Chinese Government as a university medical school, and the absolute charter granted by the Regents of the University of the State of New York, involved an obligation to maintain minimum levels of equipment, personnel and operating funds. Observance or abandonment of these "basic standard levels" could be determined only by the Board and as a considered matter of policy.

He pointed out that the institution was carrying on "three interdependent performances of very different character in themselves, but each one necessary to the work as a whole—schools, hospital, and physical plant." Upkeep of the physical plant could be determined with accuracy, and was a firm figure not subject to significant reduction. The hospital furnished "somewhat more scope for give-and-take in the matter of money. It may be extravagantly done, or... so niggardly... that it becomes inadequate for educational purposes." Changes in the Schools of Medicine and Nursing, while maintaining the levels of performance in the CMB memorandum of January 1936, were being carefully studied but changes particularly in the expensive items of foreign personnel could be made only as the nature of contracts, some extending into the years ahead, would permit.

It appeared to him that there were three alternatives open to the China Medical Board if the Trustees of The Rockefeller Foundation should feel they no longer could meet the gap between the CMB income and the College operating budget.

1. *Acceptance of educational levels lower than those then being followed.*
   Should a lowering of educational levels be decided upon, "it must not be furtive in the doing." The Ministry of Education in Nanking and the Regents of the University of the State of New York should be so

122

informed promptly, since this would affect both Chinese registration and the charter. Funds would have to be provided for early liquidation of many contracts, Chinese as well as Western, with members of the faculty who would not care to continue in an institution of lower professional standards even if their salaries were covered. "The burden of change... must fall upon the School of Medicine, for the physical plant is practically a fixed expense, and the hospital only slightly less so."

2. *Closing out temporarily*. In his judgment this would be unsound "for it would leave useless and exposed a great investment;... would shatter beyond resumption the program that has gone on successfully for a decade and a half." In addition there would be serious political repercussions; "in Chinese eyes it would be a withdrawal in the face of Japanese pressure, and a betrayal of American friendship and goodwill toward China. I don't believe the Foundation could afford the results of a step like that."

3. *A middle course*. This would mean proceeding "somewhat as at present, attempting to find the lowest costs of operation consistent with our obligations under the charters and other undertakings" but to speed up the time when the necessary changes might become effective. After remarking that it was not easy to hurry "the process of contraction and deflation" in an institution whose various elements were locked together in such a way that nothing can be dealt with piecemeal, but only as a whole, he warned that a school conducted on even such a basis would certainly cost more than the $343,000 reckoned as CMB current income, and hazarded a guess that it would cost "more than $600,000."

He concluded that even though his comments might seem "special pleading" he was "trying to look upon this extremely interesting and important undertaking without bias" and was "prepared to move in whatever direction the policy of the Board demands."

When Mr. Fosdick received this letter, he passed it on to Mr. Vincent who commented that this "excellent statement" raised several questions in his mind:

1. Is not PUMC the fundamental contribution of the RF to China?
2. Is not quality of work essential to success? Better scuttle than mediocrity.

123

3. Should not all RF resources, if they are to be limited in China, be concentrated on PUMC rather than divided between it and other programs?

In these few words, Mr. Vincent summed up the basic ideas on the PUMC shared over the years by Dr. Pearce, Dr. Gregg, Mr. Greene, and Dr. Houghton—but the official attitude of The Rockefeller Foundation and the CMB was fixed on the goal of economy. On July 1, Mr. Lobenstine, who had been elected a member and Trustee of the CMB in 1935, succeeded Mr. Vincent as Chairman of the China Medical Board. On that same day he met with Mr. Rockefeller, 3rd, and Dr. G. Canby Robinson "to consider the important question of the future financing of the PUMC, in view of the shrinkage of the income from the $12,000,000 endowment of the CMB" and of clear indications from The Rockefeller Foundation that it was not in a position "in view of its other commitments to continue making annually such large grants as in recent years" or to offer "any hope of a sufficiently large additional capital grant from the Foundation to meet the situation."

Dr. Houghton's earlier warning to the members of the Survey Commission that reduced costs must take precedence over quality of program had been taken seriously, resulting finally in a budget framework which seemed to him both "practicable and safe." He described it to Mr. Lobenstine as "a grievous disappointment to some of the men who voted for it" and anticipated that it would "shock most of the faculty," but he hoped the same "fine spirit of loyalty and cooperation" showed by the Commission members would be reflected in the total faculty.

The first ten days of September saw the Commission as a whole meeting almost daily, ending with a meeting on September 11 with an extended discussion of the form of motion by which the report should be recommended to the Trustees. They wished to be certain it was understood that in presenting proposals for a reduced budget covering a curtailed program, they were not in favor of either. The preamble and resolution as finally approved made this abundantly clear:

WHEREAS, the original terms of reference of this Commission, as established by the Trustees of the College for the purpose of implementing the objectives laid down in the memorandum of the China Medical Board, have been modified by subsequent instructions from the Board of Trustees as communicated in a letter from the Chairman of the Executive Committee under date of June 27, 1936, therefore, be it

RESOLVED that the proposals now before the Commission be approved and recommended to the Trustees, as a practicable program based on the restricted resources which are available, rather than as the statement of a program at the conservative level originally asked for, and that the original proposals as presented by the individual departments and committees concerned be filed as a part of the permanent record of this Commission.

Having served the purpose for which it had been organized, the Commission thereupon was dissolved.

Two weeks later, on September 23, 1936, Dr. Houghton presented the report to the PUMC Trustees at a Special Meeting called to consider the findings of the Survey Commission. In a seven-page introduction, he called attention to the salient features of the recommendations of the subcommittees. The most significant changes proposed were: (1) in the general administrative structure of the whole institution and (2) sharp revisions downward to arrive at a "stabilized" budget which placed operating costs "as low as compatible with safety." The administrative proposals called for a streamlining of the whole administration under a Governing Council (the Director as chairman ex-officio), functioning through three divisions: Educational Division (responsible for both the Medical School and the School of Nursing); Medical Services Division (responsible for the Hospital and for the Urban and Rural Health Stations); and Business Division "to assist the Director in the administration of the College except in matters reserved to other divisions of the Governing Council." The Medical and Nursing Faculties as such had the single function of conferring degrees, awarding diplomas, prizes and scholarships in the Medical School and School of Nursing. Their former administrative responsibilities were placed under the Educational Division which would be made up of representatives of both faculties.

The Stabilized Budget which had been worked out showed a substantial reduction of the net operating budget to US$573,047 as against that for 1935-36 which totaled US$727,258. The major part of this reduction was posited on: (1) replacement of Western personnel with US dollar salaries, by Chinese with local currency salaries, and (2) a downward revision of the salary scale. Transition to the new plan would have to be "gradual and natural," particularly in changes of academic posts and salaries which would be made only as positions were vacated by expiry of appointment, resignation or transfer. No demotion either in rank or salary was contemplated. This meant that the process of putting all the recommendations of the Commission into effect would cover several years, since the College had contractual commitments extending beyond 1940.

Each section of the report was reviewed by the Trustees in detail. During the discussion, certain agreements were reached and when these involved textual changes in the reports as presented, the necessary changes were made there and then. Two of the most significant changes dealt with the admission standards and the continued use of English as the basic language of instruction in the School of Nursing, and made clear the fact that the Trustees were sympathetic with the Dean and Nursing Faculty who were strong advocates of higher standards in nursing education.

At the conclusion of the five-hour long discussion, the report of the Survey Commission was "approved in principle as a basis for the future conduct of the College," and was referred to the CMB "for comment in the light of the objectives set forth by that body in the memorandum to the Trustees of the College, and for information as to the availability of funds to carry on the work of the College at the proposed level." The budget for 1936-37 was unaffected by the figures set down in the Stabilized Budget, but the Trustees instructed the officers to prepare the budget for 1937-38 "along the general lines of the Stabilized Budget, with the understanding that all current posts and salaries shall remain unchanged as long as present appointments continue or as long as present appointees hold these posts."

On November 24, 1936, the report of the Survey Commission and the recommendations of the Trustees which Dr. Houghton had brought from Peking, were taken up by the China Medical Board. The figures presented by Dr. Houghton showed the "stabilized" figure for the Operating Budget plus the usual annual special US dollar appropriations for commutation allowances, fellowships, visiting professors and travel abroad, and in addition the administrative budget for the China Medical Board:

PUMC

Operating budget
CS$1,638,115 at 3.2·······················	$511,942	
US$ expenses·····························	61,105	$573,047
Commutation·······························		50,000
Fellowships·································		32,000
Visiting Professors·························		25,000
Travel Abroad·····························		20,000
		$700,047

126

CMB Administration

New York Office	30,000	
Peking Office	28,000	
Reserve for depreciation of buildings and equipment		25,000
Repairs, alterations, etc., in buildings and equipment		10,000
Insurance on buildings and equipment	7,000	
		$100,000
		$800,047

Although realizing that it would take some years to come down to the level of the Stabilized Budget, the CMB clearly felt that important steps had been taken toward this goal, and received the report with "appreciation." They expressed the belief that the objectives of the College as recorded in the joint agreement on the functions of the CMB and its relations to the Trustees of the PUMC could be achieved within the general plan outlined in the report, and commended to the Trustees of the College "such further action in general conformity with the reports as appears to them to be desirable."

Present at this meeting of the CMB was Mr. Sohtsu G. King, Chairman of the Executive Committee of the PUMC Trustees, who had made a special trip from England to attend. He was familiar with the institution and its problems, and having participated in the Trustees' discussion in September he was able to add illuminating comments to the formal language of the resolutions. In response to a statement by Mr. King that the Trustees would welcome any comments and suggestions in regard to the report that the CMB might make, a committee, consisting of Dr. Alfred E. Cohn, Dr. G. Canby Robinson and Dr. Houghton, was asked, in association with Dr. Gregg, to study the report of the Survey Commission and to make to the Board such suggestions and recommendations for changes in accordance with the general plan outlined in the report as might seem to them desirable.

With the Stabilized Budget an officially accepted goal, the CMB now felt in a position to present a formal request to The Rockefeller Foundation for an appropriation to supplement CMB income in support of the College for a five-year period, rather than the annual requests of the past three years. After a careful review of estimates showing steadily decreasing expenditures and anticipated annual CMB income somewhat higher than had been feared, the request was for $2,000,000, "toward the maintenance of the PUMC during the five-year period July 1, 1937, to June 30, 1942... with the understanding that any balance unexpended at the end of this period shall be applicable to the maintenance of the College for the period July 1, 1942, to June 30, 1943." On December 16, 1936, The Rockefeller Foundation approved this request, noting that since anything left for 1942-43 would probably be insufficient for that year's needs, the Foundation would be prepared at that time to consider a further request. Mr. Fosdick's understanding of the problems of the CMB and the PUMC shows clearly in that sympathetic action.

Chapter IV

THE CHANGING SCENE

1937-1939

W<small>HEN</small> the Trustees appointed the three-man Administrative Committee to take over the direction of the College from Mr. Greene on July 1, 1935, for one year, this was obviously a temporary expedient. Everyone wanted an able Chinese Director who could devote all his time and energies to the job, but no one suitable was presently available. Dr. J. Heng Liu who had held the *pro forma* title of Director since May 1929 in order to meet Chinese government regulations, was eminently qualified for the substantive post, but was prevented by his responsibilities as head of the National Health Administration in Nanking from serving in anything but name.

The Administrative Committee proved admirably successful in keeping the institution running smoothly. All things considered, it was concluded that the continuance of the Administrative Committee was the best solution for a second year. Dr. Maxwell, Dr. R. K. S. Lim and Dr. Wu Hsien were accordingly reappointed for the year 1936-37.

As the Survey Report took shape, it was clear that its implementation in terms of personnel and budget was going to be a formidable administrative task for several years. This was naturally a matter of serious concern to the staff and a subject of much informal discussion, especially in view of the fact that Dr. Maxwell, Chairman of the Administrative Committee, was due to reach retirement age in the summer of 1937.

Out of these discussions developed a consensus that it would be in the best interests of the College if, during the two or three years of adjustment to the report of the Survey Commission, Dr. Houghton could serve as Acting Director. On December 4 the Committee of Professors unanimously recommended this to the Trustees, pointing out that "Dr. Henry S. Houghton's knowledge of the development of the College from its earliest years, his familiarity with the special circumstances of the environment in which the College carries on its work, his intimate connection with the Survey Commission, his experience in medical school administration in the United States, the respect which he commands to a high degree from the staff of the College and from its founders and supporters in the United States, all eminently fit him to direct the College during the period of transition."

This recommendation met with a favorable response from the Trustees who themselves had felt for some time that Dr. Houghton was the best man to help strengthen mutual understanding and confidence with the CMB and The Rockefeller Foundation in this period of increasing financial limitations. The China Medical Board agreed in principle to the request of the Trustees that Dr. Houghton be made available for appointment as Vice Director of the PUMC, but left it to him to say if he was agreeable to the proposal. Personally, Dr. Houghton would have preferred not to be involved in the day-by-day administration of the College, but after assuring himself on his return to Peking from New York in early March that he could count on the wholehearted support of the Trustees and of the greater part of the staff, he accepted the appointment to serve as Vice Director for three years beginning July 1, 1937, with an expression of his desire to serve the College in whatever way he could be of the greatest help. He followed this by formally resigning the Directorship of the CMB as of June 30, 1937, a step with which the CMB was in full accord. While Vice Director, he would be answerable solely to the Trustees of the PUMC.

During the spring, before assuming his College responsibilities, Dr. Houghton was engaged in consultations and conferences in Shanghai and Nanking on the question of the PUMC's role in a national program of postgraduate education. There were also important discussions affecting the program of the School of Nursing which on January 14, 1937 had been authorized by the Ministry of Education to be reorganized as a Special (Chuan Shou) School. Nine of the leading graduates of the School of Nursing participated in the discussions about the School and its program. Seven of these were in posts of importance in other institutions and two on the PUMC nursing faculty. Other participants were the Secretary of the Commission on Medical Education (Dr. C. K. Chu, a PUMC graduate); Miss Hodgman, Dean of the PUMC School of Nursing; the three members of the PUMC Administrative Committee and Dr. Houghton. Agreement was reached in principle on a basic nursing program of three years for graduates of senior middle schools and, in addition, a graduate course for those competent to enter fields of teaching or administration.

One gratifying event that spring was the formal opening of the National Medical College of Shanghai and the newly formed Shanghai Medical Center of which it was a part. The annual conference of the Chinese Medical Association had been scheduled to coincide with this event and twenty-three members of the PUMC faculty, together with Dr. Houghton, were in Shanghai to participate in the sessions of the association and to attend the ceremonies at the National Medical College. The fact that the land on which the new buildings were placed had been bought with the proceeds of the property originally purchased by The Rockefeller Foundation for the projected "Shanghai Medical School" which did not materialize, and of which Dr. Houghton had been slated to be the Director, made his presence at this occasion especially fortunate. In addition Dr. F. C. Yen, who was inaugurated as Director of the Medical Center and Dean of the Medical College, had served as Vice Director of the PUMC during the year 1927-28 when the military situation had forced the closing of the Hsiang-Ya Medical College in Changsha. This was one of many instances where the PUMC could justly take satisfaction in new institutions largely staffed by PUMC graduates and former faculty. The outreach in China that was one of the original aims of the founders was more and more visible.

As far as the Medical School was concerned, the question was whether or not the College should apply for official recognition as a Medical Postgraduate Institute, under general regulations laid down by the Ministry of Education. In relation to program, such registration would create no problems since it would be essentially securing formal approval of what was already being done in most of the teaching departments of the College. The Minister of Education in the course of a conversation with Dr. Houghton went so far as to say that the Ministry would be glad to make an appropriation toward the cost of the program. Dr. Houghton replied that since no increased cost to the regular operating budget was anticipated, it might be better to apply the government funds available for stipends to advanced workers recommended to the College by the Ministry. Dr. Houghton personally felt that it would be unwise to accept appropriations toward running expenses from the government, because of the dangers of political control or interference. He believed that freedom of policy and action in educational matters must be fully safeguarded.

In subsequent discussions in the Committee of Professors, some members of the faculty, chiefly among the Westerners, were strongly opposed to the proposed registration for fear that even without financial support, it opened the way for government interference and attempted control. Dr. Houghton himself felt that as long as it was only a matter of registration, there should be no greater difficulty than the College had experienced in the years since its registration with the Ministry. Special faculty committees studied the whole situation intensively. On June 19, 1937, the Committee of Professors in one of the final meetings before its functions would be absorbed into the new Educational Division on July 1, approved a memorandum to the Ministry of Education accepting "the invitation of the Ministry of Education for formal registration of its Graduate School of Medicine." After setting forth formal answers to questions on physical equipment, qualifications of faculty, size of budget, facilities for instruction and fields of instruction, the memorandum concluded with the following statement: "In submitting this application for registration, we wish to record our conviction, in which we are sure the Ministry will concur, that true graduate work in medicine requires the greatest possible degree of freedom and elasticity." The plan unfortunately was never tried out. In less than a month, Japanese military control of North China was complete and cooperation with the Ministry of Education of the National Government was no longer possible.

Administrative Restructuring

On July 1, Dr. Houghton was to assume the post of Acting Director; the new Bylaws would become effective on that date; preparations for setting up the new administrative structure had to be made so that the transition might go smoothly. These were busy days and weeks.

In accepting appointment, Dr. Houghton had stipulated that there be a Chinese academic Dean in his administration, a post provided for in the Bylaws but unfilled since 1929. To facilitate the setting up of the new administrative bodies, the Committee of Professors on June 17, 1937, convening for the last time, nominated Dr. C. E. Lim to this post for the year beginning July 1, 1937. The final action of the Committee was the appointment on a part-time basis of Mr. Arthur Rugh of Yenching University to the Department of Religious and Social Work, to take responsibility for the Sunday services in the College auditorium. Convinced though he was as to the importance of this department and the necessity of its continuance, Dr. Houghton in the two years since Mr. Hayes completed his term of service had been no more successful than Mr. Greene in finding a suitable person as full-time Secretary for Religious and Social Work.

Thursday, July 1, came and the new administration was ready. On Tuesday, July 6, the Governing Council held its organizing meeting, followed immediately by a similar meeting of the Educational Division at which the functions of the Director and the Dean were spelled out. The next day saw the organization of the other two divisions of the Council—the Medical Services Division and the Business Division. The administrative machinery within the College began to move according to the new pattern.

Outside the College, other forces were also moving. Wednesday, July 7, 1937 was the day of the Marco Polo Bridge "Incident"—Lukouchiao—when Japanese troops directly attacked and overwhelmed a Chinese garrison southwest of Peking. This humiliating event, remembered as the "double-seventh," marked the beginning of the Sino-Japanese War. From that moment on, the Japanese were the dominant factor in North China.

There was no immediate disruptive effect on the College. Writing to Mr. Lobenstine on July 16, Dr. Houghton first reported that the internal transition "seems to have been made easily and with little if any rippling of administrative waters." He then spoke of the Lukouchiao incident as "distressing but not particularly surprising" and one which would result in what he euphemistically described as a "greater degree of separation of Hopei (Province) from the National Government.... There is no local danger to be apprehended, as far as I can see... No long continued interruption of communications is likely to take place... and I look to see reasonably normal conditions of life resumed here before long... We have taken measures to see that supplies of essential materials are on hand. We have coal in our bunkers for something over two months firing; of rice and other staple foods, we can manage about the same period of time.... The hospital is functioning as usual, and everyone appears to be calm, although... the situation in the long run is a grave one. I do not anticipate any particular dislocation of our regular program... The discussions we have been having with the Council on Medical Education about graduate training have naturally been interfered with, and doubtless will have to be postponed until the general political landscape is clearer, but there is no particular change of purpose or policy."

One of the changes in academic organization which went into effect on July 1 called for the appointment of department heads by the Director on recommendation of the Educational Division. Hitherto, headship of a department had been an integral part of many of the full professorial appointments. To conform to the new Bylaws, while safeguarding all other terms of existing indeterminate appointments, the Trustees instructed the immediate cancellation of indeterminate contracts in accordance with the stipulated formal notice of two years, and the offer, instead, of new appointments similar in all respects except for mention of departmental headship. At the same time, the Trustees, conscious that the lowered level of the Stabilized Budget was a primary goal, appointed a group of senior Chinese professors to study the possible reduction of the number of "foreign" personnel on U.S. dollar salaries, and to report back to the Trustees.

This group (Dr. George Y. Char, Dr. C. E. Lim, Dr. R. K. S. Lim and Dr. Wu Hsien) under the chairmanship of Dr. Houghton, reviewed the academic departments one by one, noting instances where it might be possible before too long to replace Western personnel with Chinese already on the staff. In doing so, they made it plain that they were, nevertheless, in full accord with the policy adopted by the Trustees of the College and the CMB, and that "association with the world sources of science" should continue to be maintained "through the retention of a proportion of foreigners." The report concluded with the specific recommendation that "every effort should be made to have constantly either a permanent or visiting foreign professor in at least one of the divisions of the following principal fields: Physiological Sciences; Pathological Sciences; Medicine including the medical specialties; Surgery including the surgical specialties and ophthalmology; Obstetrics and Gynecology; Public Health."

Of the eleven indeterminate professional appointments in effect, six were held by "foreigners," five by Chinese, and all but one included headship of a department or division. The ten men holding appointments as "professor and head" were each duly notified that these were cancelled, "effective immediately, subject to your acceptance of a new contract now offered to you."

While the report of the committee on foreign professional staff had been adopted without question by the Executive Committee, there was certainly uneasiness among non-Chinese members of the faculty as to their own professional future and the effect of the continued emphasis on budget reduction on the quality of the College. Dr. F. R. Dieuaide chose not to accept an appointment on the new basis, but to continue to serve as Professor of Medicine and Head of the Department for 1937-38, with a final year's leave of absence in accordance with the terms of his original indeterminate appointment. Dr. H. B. Van Dyke, Professor of Pharmacology, and Dr. Peter C. Kronfeld, Professor of Ophthalmology, accepted the new appointments offered but each left within the next year for more assured futures in the United States. The three others affected, Dr. A. B. D. Fortuyn, Professor of Anatomy, Dr. R. J. C. Hoeppli, Professor of Parasitology, and Dr. Harold H. Loucks, Professor of Surgery, accepted the new indeterminate appointments as did the five Chinese professors. In due course, all whose original appointments had included headship of a department or division were so continued on recommendation of the Educational Division, but the principle had been established that the various "headships" should not be permanently limited to a few individuals.

The College was as yet so undisturbed by the political and military developments of recent days that on July 13, on recommendation of Dr. Houghton and the newly-appointed Dean, Dr. C. E. Lim, a Planning Committee was appointed consisting of Dr. Houghton, Chairman, and five Chinese professors, Dr. Char, Dr. C. E. Lim, Dr. R. K. S. Lim, Dr. C. U. Lee and Dr. Wu Hsien, for the purpose of examining all proposals for cooperation with outside organizations, whether governmental or private; to explore possibilities for enlisting interest and support for activities outside the limits of the stabilized budget; and in consultation with the heads of departments concerned to make detailed recommendations to the Educational Division. Dr. C. K. Chu, Secretary of the Commission on Medical Education, and Dr. John B. Grant, Field Director of the International Health Division of The Rockefeller Foundation, were asked to serve as advisors to the Planning Committee.

New Political Problems

The comparative quiet following the Marco Polo Bridge incident was soon succeeded by a period of tension and anxiety, with communications of all sorts interrupted. Dr. Houghton himself was caught in Tientsin when the trains stopped running; tried to reach Peking by car along with the correspondent of the *New York Times* only to find the road at Tung-hsien blocked by a Japanese bombardment, which forced their return to Tientsin until the first train, on August 4, made the usual three-hour run to Peking in nine hours. While in Tientsin, Dr. Houghton's only communication with the College was through direct radio between the American Embassy and the American Consulate General.

There was great anxiety in New York for the welfare of the staff, but by July 30, messages to The Rockefeller Foundation, sent through the State Department in Washington from the Embassy in Peking and from the Foundation's Shanghai office, gave reassurance that the institution was functioning normally, morale was good, everybody was safe—"no cause for anxiety." There still were doubts in New York as to the wisdom of members of the staff in the United States proceeding to Peking as planned, resulting in cancelled sailings by the China Medical Board. In Peking four younger Chinese members of the staff, all PUMC graduates, were waiting to start for the United States under fellowships granted by the Trustees; the passport office in Tientsin had been blown to pieces during the recent bombardment, no trains were running south, and very few boats. The prospects were not encouraging but the group finally left Peking on August 11—squeezing into cars where every seat had been occupied hours before the scheduled departure time and virtually no standing room was left for the ride to Tientsin. From there they would go to Shanghai by boat as deck passengers along with four hundred fortunate others out of the ten thousand waiting for passage south.

Postal and telegraphic communications continued to be uncertain and greatly delayed. In the meantime the hospital was functioning as usual and preparations were being made to open the academic year on September 9 as scheduled. Many who had gone home for the summer might find it impossible to return, but any on hand on that date would find classes open. Special arrangements would be made to help late arrivals catch up on lectures, laboratory and clinical work which they had missed.

The complete takeover of Peking which followed the entry of Japanese troops into the city on August 4, 1937, left the College in a thoroughly anomalous situation. All but two of the Trustees were in eastern or central China and to all intents and purposes, inaccessible and unavailable for meetings; one of the two in North China was preparing to leave as soon as possible. Dr. Houghton had to face the fact that there would then be not even a quorum of the Executive Committee to whom to refer matters for final decision. After consultation with the two available Trustees, one of whom was Mr. Lin Hsin-kwei, the College's counsel, Dr. Houghton took two emergency steps: (1) at the American Embassy he registered the China Medical Board as an American corporation, filing a statement of the Board's local assets; and (2) he personally assumed complete charge of the College and its plant on behalf of the owners.

On August 18, he reported to the whole Governing Council on "the state of emergency" in which the College was now functioning and the need for calm and careful adjustment to the existing conditions. The emergency measures would prevail only until the Trustees could resume their normal functions on behalf of the institution. No basic change of status was contemplated. He himself would remain in Peking as long as existing conditions continued, without making his previously planned trip to New York. Rising prices of foodstuffs were being carefully watched and if this situation should become much worse, steps would be taken to relieve the resulting pressure on employees in the lower wage brackets. It was important to maintain normal routines so as to have the minimum interference with the educational program of the institution.

The Business Division opened a branch office of the College in Tientsin with Mr. Bradfield in charge, to help staff and students passing through Tientsin who might be exposed to delay or even detention by the military. In addition he could look after shipments, handle purchases, and represent the College in any of the unforeseen circumstances that might arise while the dislocation of communications continued.

New Inter–Board Tensions

In the midst of this turbulent situation, Dr. Houghton received a letter from Mr. Lobenstine, which had been written on June 30, before the situation in Peking had flared up. This dealt among other things with a letter from Dr. Houghton written on May 18, after the conversations in Nanking with the Ministry of Education about the PUMC graduate program, and the suggestion from the Minister of possible government subsidy. Mr. Lobenstine also touched on a letter from Dr. Houghton dated June 3, wherein he had mentioned the hoped-for time "when the College can be consistently operated over a long period at an outlay not exceeding US$800,000 annually and fixed provision has been made for this sum."

Mr. Lobenstine had referred both these letters to Mr. Rockefeller, 3rd for information as he frequently did, this being especially easy since Mr. Rockefeller's office and that of the CMB were both located in the RCA building. Sometimes such letters were returned without comment. This time Mr. Lobenstine was called in for conference. Mr. Rockefeller was disturbed lest Dr. Houghton's response to the Minister of Education might endanger the chances of future offers of governmental support, "when such support is the one main source which it appears can be looked to for any substantial financial help in China." Mr. Lobenstine also reported to Dr. Houghton that Mr. Rockefeller did not want it assumed that fixed and indeterminate provision of the sum of US$800,000 a year had already been made, when actually all that had been guaranteed was a subsidy to the CMB of $2,000,000 spread over a five or six-year period. If $800,000 were to be considered the "permanent and fixed level of operations" this might result in a slackening of economies on the part of the College administrators and staff.

At the same time as Mr. Lobenstine's letter reached Peking, a cable came from New York reporting that, contrary to Dr. Houghton's advice, the sailings of two American professors had been cancelled. Dr. Houghton was not happy with either the cable or letter, replying by cable that "as a matter of principle and procedure it seems to me that recommendations from here should not be reversed in New York without consultation."

Dr. Houghton devoted the next two days to two long letters to Mr. Lobenstine. In the first of these, after pointing out "the fact that the College is now being conducted in occupied territory which will be politically reorganized before long puts an entirely new complexion upon our relation to government and to indigenous support," he went on to the principles underlying his having declined the proposal by the Minister of Education "to put fifty thousand silver dollars into the operating funds of the College. My answer is that I do not propose to sell out the freedom of this institution and the maintenance of its scientific and educational standards for a contribution amounting to less than two percent of our annual upkeep. When the Government becomes a financial partner it immediately begins to mold institutional policies and practices to its own particular pattern. I have watched that occurring in all of the other private universities that have accepted Government subsidy, and definitely decided against it... the Chairman of the Board of Trustees was... in full sympathy with my reluctance to have Government participation in the operating budget." Dr. Houghton then turned to the matter of stabilization for a long period at approximately $800,000. "During the past two years, we have reduced operation costs by approximately $250,000 in a total of $900,000 ($897,907). This is a staggering sum to cut out of maintenance, and of course you will understand that under the new conditions the College cannot be what it was... In spite of the changes that have been made in the College, it is still, I think, a good medical school. But it has been pared down to the last cent. The difference between the operating budget of 1935-36... and that estimated for 1938-39... represents not only the application of practicable and desirable economies pressed as far as we dare, but also a margin applied to a wide and diversified range of scientific studies, all of which have their effect upon the professorial life of the institution, and go to the making of a significant school of medicine. This margin you have given up; to cut more off will destroy even a claim to educational worthiness." He concluded by warning that it was not too early to be "pondering the situation even now, for if marked changes in the status of the College are to be made in 1942 they will need long preparation."

Having made his position clear for the official record in relatively restrained language, he felt free to set down in his second letter, marked *personal and confidential*, "remarks somewhat more intimate and pungent." He wished "absolutely without personal animus, and in an entirely cheerful spirit" to make no further arguments but "largely to blow off steam to you privately and to ask some questions." At the outset, he said that "if it were not for this confounded (and wholly artificial) war, I should be preparing to leave for New York in the autumn with no expectation of returning to China. For to be quite bald about it, I have not the slightest interest in the prospect which your letter holds out... As it is, of course, I shall not leave here until peaceful conditions are assured, and until a comparatively smooth path ahead can be seen. My business is to maintain good morale and to keep the College going steadily until we are quite out of the woods." After discussing briefly how long the current political and military "disturbance" might last, he returned to his main theme: "What I am impatient about is this confounded puttering with the PUMC. Why not face the situation realistically, for once? If the RF doesn't want to keep it going, even at the bottom level of educational decency, why in heaven's name don't they give it away?... It is this idea that somehow you can eat your cake and still have it that strains my serenity. You can't have a good school without spending the money that it costs. And when I say you cannot run a first class medical school here for less than $800,000 a year, and that you cannot let governments in China monkey with it without damaging the works beyond repair, I know what I am talking about. It is a crux,... that calls for a clear-cut decision; either one thing or the other should be done. What your letter proposes, however, is to muddle, perhaps in the hope that the momentum of the College's great name (honestly earned) will carry it along even though in reality it is only a shell and a whited sepulchre. That, I'm sure you will agree, would be educationally immoral... With the substance of what you set before me... if it truly represents the Board's views, I find myself almost wholly out of agreement. Let me put the thing, as far as I am concerned, into one-two-three order:

1. I think the RF should in due course add about eight million from capital to the CMB endowment, so as to return an annual income of approximately (at four percent) eight hundred thousand dollars.

2. If this is out of the question, they should consider whether they are prepared to carry on indefinitely at the minimum level for a good school, by periodic supplementary grants.

3. If they are determined to taper off, it is important for me to know it, so I can try to find something else to do. In saying this I am quite certain that I speak for all of the principal foreigners and Chinese connected with it. No one of them will want to go on in a place for which they have to blush.

4. If they want to make some disposition of the place to government or to a

private organization, I am wiling to help find alternative possibilities, but not of course to maintain any connection with it.

"These four paragraphs may serve as my creed, if you like; so you will see how necessary it is for me to have the issues clearly faced. These words are for your private eye and ear, of course. If you wish to do so, however, you may show them to RBF [Raymond B. Fosdick], who is a good friend and a wise owl."

Once again, in unequivocal terms, the philosophy of Buttrick, Welch, Simon Flexner, Franklin McLean, Richard Pearce, George Vincent, Roger Greene, Alan Gregg, and Henry Houghton had been cogently argued against the recurrent counsels for economy for its own sake.

Dr. Houghton's "personal and confidential" letter of August 20 reached Mr. Lobenstine on September 22, the "official" one of August 19 not arriving until October 3, along with letters of August 5, 6, 12, 17 and September 10. Such were the difficulties of attempting any kind of effective communication. Cables and radiograms were no better. For the most part, the only sure route was the American Embassy radio, a courtesy extended for matters of importance but subject to the Embassy's own rules and regulations, sometimes resulting in unsigned and incomprehensible messages.

Mr. Lobenstine was understandably distressed at Dr. Houghton's reaction and under the circumstances regretted that he had ever written. On September 30 he replied in a conciliatory tone reporting that Mr. Fosdick believed there had been no change in the attitude of the CMB or the Foundation, and was confident that the current grant would be succeeded by "satisfactory plans" for the institution's future. Mr. Fosdick also cabled and wrote in the same vein. As far as Dr. Houghton was concerned, the situation was satisfactorily closed—at least for the time being.

For the PUMC, as for all of North China, the rest of 1937 was filled with uncertainties. On September 9 the College administration informed all American citizens on the staff that anyone who wished to follow the State Department's advice that they should consider leaving China while facilities for doing so were available, would be permitted to terminate his services without prejudice to contractual privileges or obligations. Not one member of the professional staff took advantage of this.

At the same time, great pressure was being exerted on both senior and junior Chinese faculty members to join civilian or military governmental agencies outside North China organizing resistance against the Japanese.

A considerable number found their way through the lines to take up positions in medical and health agencies operating in Free China. Others, returning from study abroad, were diverted to government service on arrival in Shanghai or Hong Kong and did not get back to the College.

Dr. Houghton sympathized with those who went west, but he had no idea of any voluntary closing of the PUMC, saying that he could see no reason that anyone should "apologize for the existence of the PUMC here, just because the Japanese forces had invaded the place. We have far more real right to be here than they, and I propose to go right along with the job, quietly and pleasantly, unless and until we are forcibly stopped... then, of course, we should have to close up shop; not without a big squawk, however, loud enough to be heard pretty well around the world." And again: "If the College was designed to help the Chinese to be a lighthouse, not only of science and skill but of humanitarian service and spiritual leadership, it would be appalling to have its work falter at this time. The staff members, foreign and Chinese alike are here, eager and ready to carry the responsibilities and burdens that have to be carried; the students... are crowding in from everywhere... These young people are looking to us for help and encouragement, and we cannot let them down... Thus far, we have been receiving consideration, aid and courtesy from all sides in carrying on our normal program."

The gaps left by the members of the faculty who did not return to Peking were not easy to fill, but those who stayed on, Chinese and Western alike, recognizing the importance of the institution to the morale and stability of the entire community, gave themselves wholeheartedly to their work.

On September 9, the Medical School reopened with 65% of its students in attendance. Others filtered in as the weeks went by, arriving singly and in small groups by devious and hazardous routes. By late October, 93 out of a possible 110 medical students had enrolled, along with a number of guest students cut off from their home schools. The School of Nursing was full, vacancies in the entering class having been filled by promising young women prevented from leaving Peking for study abroad or elsewhere in China. The house staff of the hospital was complete. Graduate students numbered 69. Dr. Houghton reported "an admirable spirit of earnestness to get on with their training, and the utmost eagerness to learn all they can. We are doing our best... not only in sustaining their instruction, but also in maintaining a high morale among them."

In a report dated October 20, which went to the scattered Trustees "by discreet hands," Dr. Houghton, with cautious understatement, gave an admirable summary of the situation in these precarious days when the responsibility for decisions rested on him alone. He spoke of the difficulty of the situation for the staff, particularly the younger men, who chafed under life in an occupied area and were troubled because they were doing nothing of a direct and tangible nature for their country. Late in July in response to a circular telegram from the Ministry of Education, a group of twenty-eight doctors and nurses volunteered for such services as might be called for, and this information was sent to the Ministry. Nothing further was heard from the Ministry, however, and by the first of September it was no longer possible for them to leave Peking openly. The only way had been to give anyone desiring to go an indeterminate leave of absence, each one making whatever arrangements he could to pass through the lines.

Dr. Houghton reported to the Trustees that since he could not leave China as long as the existing state of war continued, he asked Mr. Bowen to take to New York the financial reports, budget estimates for 1938-39, and requests for miscellaneous appropriations, for submission to the CMB. Mr. Bowen left on October 25, at which time Mr. Bradfield closed the emergency Tientsin office and returned to handle the controller's and treasurer's duties at the College.

The College by this time was receiving "every consideration" from the local authorities. No indication of limitation or interference had appeared. The earlier acute problems as to supplies of coal and foodstuffs and currency had subsided. Local income, which for the first two months had dropped markedly, started rising once more. It seemed to Dr. Houghton, therefore, that "the way seems clear... for the College to maintain its status and program intact at least for as long a time as can clearly be foreseen. This is to me an important function: the removal of cultural, educational and other institutions, even when it has been necessary, has given the world an unfortunate impression of giving up without argument regions and rights that belong to China, whether the former are occupied for the time being by foreign troops or not. To do so further (any more than is absolutely necessary) appears to me to invite expropriation, and to advertise a defeatist attitude. With this point in mind, I am doing my best to keep the College on a going and productive basis, and also helping as much as possible in doing the same for other related organizations, especially the First Midwifery School, and the Geological Survey and Cenozoic Laboratory. I earnestly hope that the other members of the Board will feel that this is a sound and proper attitude to take."

And so the weeks went by, staff and students alike demonstrating amazing adaptability to the fluid and unpredictable situation around them. The academic program maintained its normal course. It was in the hospital that the external dislocation of life was most seriously felt. The number of paying patients was greatly reduced with a corresponding increase in the demand for free hospitalization and clinical services. This meant a substantial decrease in the hospital income which was so important an item in the budget. The first four months of the fiscal year compared with the same period of the previous year showed a decrease of 35% in income from in-patients and of 47% from out-patients. This was not an easy time to be budgeting on the steadily decreasing scale posited by the Survey's Stabilized Budget. That budget covered only normal peace-time activities of the institution, with no margin for unusual activities incident to war or other unsettled conditions. Mr. Bowen who had been so insistent on cutting the budget to the bone, himself commented that "extra activities ... if there are any will need to be financed from extra-budgetary sources ... appreciable reductions in costs by curtailment of activities cannot be made at short notice and without definite restatement of policy and program."

The China Medical Board accepted the budget estimates and other financial statements as recommended by Dr. Houghton, and as it was impossible to have them passed upon by the Trustees, made the necessary appropriations. Note was also taken of Dr. Houghton's actions in the existing emergency with respect to the Board's property. For his protection, should he be challenged, Dr. Houghton was formally appointed special representative of the CMB "to take such action on behalf of the Board as may seem to him necessary or advisable in connection with any question which may arise in relation to the property of the Board at Peiping, now utilized by the PUMC, if such question arises under circumstances which in the opinion of Dr. Houghton make it difficult or impossible to obtain timely instructions from the Board in regard thereto."

On January 12, 1938, three members of the PUMC Trustees Executive Committee, constituting a quorum, succeeded in meeting together in

144

Tientsin, the first official meeting of the Trustees in six months. Their first action was to ratify and approve the circular action authorizing Dr. Houghton to take complete charge of the plant and operation on behalf of the Trustees for six months as a matter of war emergency. Similar approval was given to twelve actions taken by Dr. Houghton under that authorization such as the various requests to the CMB for appropriations for 1938-39, which would normally have been brought before the Executive Committee. Since there was little likelihood of securing a quorum of Trustees on March 9, the statutory date for the Annual Meeting, they agreed that for the continued orderly administration of the College the Executive Committee should for the time being assume all the powers of the Trustees including electing members of the board and officers for the coming year. They then proceeded "subject to ratification by the full board," to the election of Trustees in the Class of 1941, officers, Executive Committee, Finance Committee and Committee on the Audit. The Executive Committee was made up of five Trustees resident in Peking. The terms of Mr. Greene and Dr. Chang Po-ling, both in the Class of 1938, were not renewed since neither was easily available for attendance at meetings or for service on the Committee.

The existence once more of a functioning Executive Committee made it possible to approve, subject to continued favorable local conditions, Dr. Houghton's request for a three-month leave of absence beginning in early March to make a quick trip to New York.

Although the doubts of getting a quorum proved well founded, on March 9 Dr. Houghton, en route to New York, was able to meet in Shanghai with five Trustees. Obviously, no formal business could be transacted, but each signed a copy of the minutes of the last meeting of the Executive Committee, which they had not attended, as evidence of concurrence in the actions taken.

While the academic year wore on in reasonably normal fashion, evidence of the abnormal situation in which the institution was operating was the decision of the Educational Division early in May that the graduation exercises would take place at a joint meeting of the Faculties of the Medical College and the School of Nursing, this meeting to be open to members of the faculties and graduating classes only. Traditionally the PUMC Commencement had been a gala public occasion with a colorful academic procession across the great white marble main court to the

Auditorium in which the Trustees and various government officials participated. No one wanted to invite representatives of the puppet regime to these exercises or to take the chance of having them appear uninvited. And so the graduation of the classes of 1938, 1939, 1940, and 1941 followed their own simple but dignified pattern: the faculties, in academic dress, meeting in formal session in the large entrance lobby of the auditorium approved the awarding of the degrees and diplomas; a student marshal then summoned the graduating classes, medical students in the distinctive PUMC regalia and nursing students in starched uniform and cap; the two deans presented the candidates to the Director who handed them their diplomas; and in less than half an hour everyone adjourned to "C" court where families and friends waited to greet the graduates.

During Dr. Houghton's absence, two occurrences pointed up other problems which the institution might be increasingly called upon to face. The first was "instructions" from the Ministry of Education of the Provisional Government to participate in the "Anti-Communist Party Suppression Campaign" during the week of June 13, complete with placards and slogans. The academic year having closed on June 10, it was possible to ignore these instructions without any direct confrontation with the authorities concerned, but the Trustees agreed with the administration that the College's established policy of non-participation in political activities of whatever nature should be maintained in any future situation. In this connection, a "searching party" of Chinese police officers and Japanese civilians appeared at the College one morning to conduct a search for communist literature. They had no credentials and the administrative officers of the College declined to permit the search unless some official document were presented. The group left without protest, returning a few hours later with an acceptable communication, and after an hour's inspection during which they were accompanied by senior administrative officers of the College, a certificate was given that no subversive material had been found (the officers of the College on their part certifying that no college property was missing as a result of the search). These events were reported to the American Embassy for information, but without any request for action by the Embassy.

A previous incident not directly affecting the College but affecting the field station at Choukoutien of the Cenozoic Laboratory for anthropological research in Asia, of which the Department of Anatomy was an integral

146

part, had occurred on May 11 when three Chinese employees of the station were executed by Japanese troops operating in that region. Such occurrences increased the underlying sense of uneasiness felt by many.

On July 15, 1938, Dr. Houghton returned to Peking, having devoted much of his two months in the United States to filling two major professorships—Medicine and Pharmacology—and also in wide-ranging discussions, especially with Dr. Gregg and Mr. Lobenstine, on internal and external problems of the PUMC. After reaching Peking, he reported that all was going well at the College "barring the general unhappiness and unrest among the younger Chinese element," and that from the point of view of political security, the institution appeared to be safe. One matter calling for action by the Executive Committee was Dr. J. Heng Liu's resignation as Director. Dr. Liu's service as titular Director since May 1, 1929, had meant much to the College, but it was recognized that for the present it might simplify the problems of dealing with "outside authorities" to accept his resignation. In so doing on July 22, 1938, the Executive Committee expressed the hope that he would "continue to have an interest in the welfare and future development of the institution with which he has had so long a connection."

Through the rest of the summer and autumn, the discussions with Dr. Gregg and Mr. Lobenstine continued through lengthy letters in which opinions were fully and frankly stated, for the most part amicably. With Mr. Lobenstine the main point at issue was the delicate one of staff morale, and the extent to which the China Medical Board should concern itself in such internal questions. Dr. Houghton acknowledged that not everyone on the staff was happy over recent changes but commented that his experiences in Iowa and later in the University of Chicago, both institutions which recently passed through a "crux of internal turmoil," had taught him not to expect immediate results. However, if Mr. Lobenstine should be troubled by anything specific he hoped he would hear from him directly about it, and that no communications would go to staff members, even if personal friends of long standing, about policies and procedures without copies being sent to Dr. Houghton for information. To this Mr. Lobenstine rather formally agreed, saying that his "official correspondence in regard to PUMC matters is naturally either with the Trustees of the College or with you as Vice Director."

In one of his letters to Mr. Lobenstine, Dr. Houghton spoke of "reactions to the changes... necessitated by financial readjustments of the past three or four years" which in some cases had been severe and directed at Dr. Houghton personally. As far as the younger Chinese were concerned, the "limitation of jobs and fixation of salaries under the stabilized budget" meant that each year more of them would have to be looking for positions elsewhere, which naturally was a cause of some anxiety for the future, but was similar to conditions existing in colleges and universities in the United States. Changes in "foreign" personnel, either on the initiative of the persons themselves or by action of the officers, also had repercussions. The loss of three senior faculty members in a period of a few months had been upsetting. "All this must be expected during these times of painful readjustment. Some degree of personal ill-will is inevitable and only time and calmness will end it." He expected that with the coming of some of the new appointees, "old animosities will gradually grow dim." He pointed out, however, that "an element of war psychology... enters into our emotional situation here. It is not only the natural tension that exists among those who are in an agony of apprehension about the outcome of the present turmoil, but the very real fact that those who stay in an occupied region for any reason whatever are likely to be objects of suspicion and resentment to their friends in the south and west." In more personal terms he wrote: "Much of what has been going on here is physiologically a part of unpleasant organizational changes. From the first I have had no illusion about the difficulties to be faced. You have indicated your uneasiness so clearly, however, that I am constrained to report fully on the situation as it appears to me." Dr. Houghton concluded these comments with "one final word. This immensely difficult job cannot be carried on successfully unless the administrator responsible for it has the confidence and backing of his superior officers. If I have not got that part of it that comes from New York, you must tell me so... I have said to you before this, that I feel you should be free to collect judgments about the state of the College from staff members if you need to do so, but I must be acquainted with the findings in due course. Otherwise I am of no use to you, or to the job." This plain speaking brought a prompt and understanding reply from Mr. Lobenstine. The tensions which had been building up in New York and in Peking were relieved for the moment.

The correspondence with Dr. Gregg dealt chiefly with what Dr. Houghton called "the triangular arrangement of Foundation, China Medical

Board and College" which in his opinion had proved unsatisfactory to all three boards. Since there seemed little likelihood under existing circumstances of his returning to New York early in 1939 for further face-to-face discussions as had been expected, he wrote at some length spelling out his views on organizational changes that should be made. Dr. Houghton felt that the China Medical Board which had been set up so as to relieve the Foundation from direct involvement in the affairs of the College, had failed to do so "and as things stand now it does nothing that could not be done as effectively (and with far less loss of motion) by the Foundation itself." He spoke of the continuing uncertainty in the minds of the PUMC Trustees as to the functions and relationships of the China Medical Board, resulting in part from "the exercise by the Board in 1934 of its charter powers of ownership. The wounds of that episode were very deep and the scars will not dissolve, I think, for a long time." On the other hand, he believed that the Trustees who had always looked upon The Rockefeller Foundation as the real source of support and the court of final appeal, would be likely to accept without resentment or suspicion the Foundation's cooperation with them through inspection and consultation on policies. Once again he mentioned the fact that throughout East Asia the College was invariably viewed as a Rockefeller Foundation activity, a circumstance which had certainly protected the institution from "persecution (or worse) in the past fifteen months and is likely to spare us acute trouble during the next few years." He concluded this analysis by stating that "the sorest spot in the triple alliance is in New York" and that a more direct way of dealing with the Foundation would be "greatly for the good of the College."

Dr. Gregg sympathized with Dr. Houghton's point of view, which he passed on to those most concerned—Mr. Fosdick, Mr. Lobenstine and Mr. Rockefeller, 3rd. There followed a number of informal conferences attended also by Dr. G. Canby Robinson and Dr. Alfred E. Cohn, the two medical members of the CMB. Dr. Robinson and Dr. Cohn, both of whom had served as Visiting Professors at the College, had come to question the value of their role on the Board, and in the light of the whole complicated network of relationships between the boards, were even considering resigning from the CMB. The consensus arrived at in these discussions was that the Foundation was not yet ready to increase the CMB endowment to a level which would enable it to support the PUMC, nor would it consider at that juncture the elimination of the CMB and resumption of direct control of the College. An immediate expedient was agreed upon—that the Foundation should transfer forthwith to the CMB the unexpended balance of the $2,000,000 which had been appropriated to supplement CMB income, thus eliminating for the next four years the annual CMB request, and putting off consideration of any long-term rearrangement of administrative relationships.

Plans were made to take formal action on this proposal at a meeting of the RF already scheduled for early December following which Mr. Rockefeller, Jr., Chairman of the Foundation Board of Trustees, would write a personal letter to Dr. Houghton reporting the action, and calling his attention to the fact that the College's relationship would hereafter be entirely with the CMB.

The Rockefeller Foundation Trustees met on December 7, 1938. The proposed letter to Dr. Houghton was already in draft before the meeting. The final text had been worked on successively by Mr. Rockefeller, 3rd, Mr. Lobenstine, and finally by Mr. Rockefeller, Jr. before he signed it. After reporting on the action turning over the balance of the $2,000,000 appropriation to the CMB, he emphasized that this action represented no change in the Foundation's interest in the college. "Rather, its purpose is to carry out the existing policy by providing for a closer and more satisfactory working relationship between the college and the China Medical Board." He then recalled the Foundation's hopes in 1928 when the $12,000,000 grant was made to the CMB together with full title to the land, buildings and equipment of the PUMC, that the Foundation should gradually withdraw from responsibility for the institution. "While it was foreseen that annual grants from the Foundation might for a number of years be necessary to supplement the income of the China Medical Board, it was frankly hoped and confidently expected that other sources, perhaps Chinese, could be found to make up the deficit. A good deal of water has, of course, gone under the bridge in the last ten years. The income on the $12,000,000 fund has fallen, and no sources other than the Foundation have been discovered to assist in maintaining the budget. Consequently, the grants from the Foundation have been continued, and for the present the situation has been taken care of, certainly through 1942. It is to be hoped that by 1941-42, when the Foundation reconsiders its pledge, the situation will have become more stabilized, and hence that it will be possible to make more specific and comprehensive plans for the future." He went on to explain that he was mentioning all this because he understood that there was some feeling in Peking that the CMB was perhaps an unnecessary organization and that it would be better if the College dealt directly with the Foundation. His personal opinion was that it would be "most unwise to consider this suggestion at the present time, if at all." Although the plans made in 1928 had not worked out as hoped, he believed that the reasons which led to these plans were still valid and that "we should adhere to our general objective of lodging the ultimate responsibility for the financing of the PUMC in an organization separately incorporated and wholly independent of the Foundation." He pointed out that the action just taken by the Trustees was in line with that point of view.

Mr. Rockefeller's letter ended with an expression of distress at hearing that Dr. Houghton had been ill and "the earnest hope that you will give yourself an unhurried opportunity for complete recovery." The illness mentioned by Mr. Rockefeller was a debilitating combination of anemia and what Dr. Houghton himself described as the "pseudo-sprue of North China" which had been troubling him since the summer. This had not kept him from carrying on his administrative responsibilities while undergoing therapy, but it did sap his energies.

Early in January 1939 it seemed to Dr. Houghton, his administrative colleagues, and the Trustees, that the local political situation had momentarily quieted down enough for him to go to New York to report to the CMB on the state of the College in its altered political environment, discuss possible future developments, and line up prospects for the visiting professor program. He accordingly left Peking on January 30 and in Shanghai attended the long-delayed Adjourned Annual Meeting of the Trustees for 1938. A quorum being present, all the emergency actions of the Executive Committee and of Dr. Houghton in the previous sixteen months were ratified and approved. Following this, Dr. Houghton sailed for New York traveling by way of Europe, the Trustees having lengthened his leave sufficiently so that his health might benefit from the long sea voyage.

He arrived in New York on March 30. Mr. Rockefeller's letter had reached Peking just as Dr. Houghton was leaving, and he deferred replying by letter in anticipation of direct discussion in New York. From the CMB office, he wrote Mr. Rockefeller that he was looking forward to seeing him in the near future, but in the meantime assuring him that "no uneasiness exists in China about the CMB as far as I know. From time to time I have myself raised questions about the scope of the Board's functions and relationships but this has solely been in the interest of trying to find the simplest and most effective way of dealing with our large and complex programs in the Orient. I thank you warmly for the generous thought that prompted so full an explanation of the purposes of the Foundation in respect to the CMB and am glad to assure you that my colleagues and I are ready to cooperate fully in meeting the Foundation's wishes." Informal discussion of the problems in which both men were so keenly interested was helpful in arriving at a clearer understanding of the factors involved.

On May 9 Dr. Houghton attended a Special Meeting of the CMB at which he reported on the political and military situation in North China, and presented the College budget for 1939-40. At this same meeting it was decided that Mr. Lobenstine should visit China during 1939-40 as a representative of the CMB, to visit not only the College but also South and West China "in order to meet the College Trustees not resident in Peiping and to secure firsthand information concerning conditions throughout the country."

Dr. Houghton meanwhile travelled about the United States lining up candidates for visiting professorships during the years ahead, and was delighted to find so many who would be prepared to accept. Writing from the steamer crossing the Pacific he commented on the plans for Mr. Lobenstine to visit China in the autumn, saying that he hoped he would plan to attend the Adjourned Annual (1939) Meeting of the Trustees in the early winter. Dr. Houghton himself wanted to talk over with Mr. Lobenstine some ideas he had about the next ten years of the College "in the terms outlined to me by Mr. Rockefeller, Jr., in our recent talks in New York."

When he reached Peking early in August 1939, Dr. Houghton found things quiet with no acute problems apparent in the College. The autumn continued smoothly but with an increasing consciousness that Peking was an occupied city and that censorship of the mails and cables called for great caution both in Peking and in New York lest some inadvertent mention of an individual in "Free China" bring trouble to his family in Peking.

Mr. Lobenstine arrived on November 13 and spent two weeks re-acquainting himself with the College and renewing old friendships before going down to Shanghai with Dr. Houghton for the Trustees' meeting. This visit had been planned in return for those of Dr. Hu Shih and Mr. Sohtsu G. King to New York the previous years. It was hoped that such exchanges between the two boards would serve to reassure the Trustees of the continuing interest and support of the CMB and would result in better understanding of common problems.

Mr. Lobenstine had no other specific instructions or commission from the CMB, but the previous summer's correspondence with Dr. Houghton notwithstanding, his personal concern about morale in the institution persisted. He accordingly embarked on a program of "personal and confidential" talks with individuals (staff and trustees, Chinese and Western) in which he seemed to be probing for complaints and grievances. Inevitably Dr. Houghton became aware of what was going on and understandably resented what he felt was an attack on himself and his administration of the College, a deliberate undermining of his position. By the time the Trustees, officers and Mr. Lobenstine assembled in Shanghai on December 4, 1939, tensions were apparent.

The Trustees were seriously disturbed by the Controller's growing tendency, especially when Dr. Houghton was away from the College, to take independent actions affecting the budget without advance consultation with either the Business Division or the Executive Committee of the Trustees, although both bodies were easily accessible at short notice. For example, a special appropriation to cover supplementary subsistence allowances for the Chinese staff on silver salaries was actually made by the CMB before the Trustees were even informed that Mr. Bowen had recommended this by cable through Dr. Houghton, although the rising cost of living was a matter about which the Trustees were greatly concerned.

An even more egregious bypassing of the Trustees had become evident at a meeting of the Executive Committee in Peking on November 20, 1939, just two weeks before the Adjourned Annual Meeting, when the Controller asked for approval of the financial report for the fiscal year 1938-39 which showed *overspendings* as of June 30, 1939, amounting to US$38,342.37 and CS$40,776.58, overspendings which had taken place without the knowledge of the Trustees. This was coupled with the proposal that the Executive Committee ask the CMB for an ex-post-facto appropriation to cover these overspendings, and to provide a further US$50,000 and CS$100,000 to cover similar requirements anticipated in the current budget for 1939-40.

The Trustees had been highly sensitized by their unhappy experiences of the early 1930's to the importance of careful budgeting and economy, and keeping expenditures within the budget limits. It came to them as a real shock that the man who had been sent from New York to ensure drastic reductions should ignore those limits. Finding that the proposed increases in the current budget had not been discussed with the Business Division, the Executive Committee referred the Controller's proposal directly to the Business Division for consideration and for a recommendation to the Trustees. (The Trustees did not know that as early as August 7, 1939, Mr. Bowen had been exchanging cables with the CMB Treasurer about the overspendings, that these had been reported at a Special Meeting of the CMB on September 28, and had been referred to the CMB Executive Committee for action as soon as definite figures and explanations should be received.) Immediately added, therefore, to the docket for the Adjourned Annual Meeting, was the Business Division's recommendation submitted through the Acting Director, for additional sums of US$50,000 and $100,000 to cover "increased costs of operation resulting from the exchange situation."

Six of the fifteen Trustees attended this meeting, one more than the quorum of five specified in a revision of the Bylaws approved by a majority of the Trustees on February 6, 1939, as an emergency measure. Dr. Houghton was there in his dual capacity as Trustee and Acting Director of the College. Following the regular practice that both financial officers should not be away from the College at the same time, Mr. Bowen had stayed in Peking while the Treasurer, Mr. Bradfield, accompanied Dr. Houghton to Shanghai.

Mr. Lobenstine was cordially welcomed by the Chairman, and responded with greetings from his CMB colleagues in New York, expressing their regard for the Trustees, their gratification at the uninterrupted operation of the College, and their appreciation of the cooperative way in which the difficult task of budget reduction had been carried out. Mentioning the continued personal interest of Mr. John D. Rockefeller, Jr., in the work of the College, he also touched on the question of the triangular relationships. He concluded with a statement of his conviction that the effective fulfillment of the aims of the founders lay not only in its academic performance but "in the firm rooting of the institution into the life of the country through a strong, effective, and independent local board of Trustees" and he pledged the support of the CMB in assisting the Trustees to achieve this desired end.

The Trustees were in a mood to be critical on the whole matter of the financial operation of the College, and they raised many questions with regard to the form of the financial statements, noting also that there had been "certain irregularities in procedure" which they asked the Acting Director to correct. They called for either periodic revisions of the budget or regular interim reports to be submitted to the Trustees, showing actual operating figures in comparison with budget estimates.

In the absence of the Controller, it fell to Dr. Houghton as Acting Director to put forward Mr. Bowen's point of view that revisions of the budget were inconsistent with the budget stabilization which was the aim of all recent measures taken. In the end, the Trustees instructed the Controller to present to them a quarterly report with detailed statements of actual operating costs in comparison with budget estimates, together with explanations covering variations from the original estimates.

When Dr. Houghton then presented the recommendation of the Business Division for an increase of the current Operating Budget, he was so well fortified by the detailed figures and analysis worked out in the recent meetings of the Division that the formal request to the CMB for the necessary US$50,000 and $100,000 was approved without reservation. The Acting Director's comprehensive report on the work of the College for the year 1938-39 was discussed with interest and warm appreciation for "the satisfactory condition of the College in spite of the difficult external circumstances."

Mr. Bowen and Mr. Bradfield were re-elected Controller and Treasurer respectively but without the specific definition of their responsibilities which Mr. Bradfield had hoped might curb Mr. Bowen's tendency to extend his activities into more and more aspects of the business and financial operation of the College, pushing the Treasurer aside.

Altogether it had not been a particularly happy meeting. Dr. Houghton returned to Peking discouraged and wondering whether he should not begin to lay his plans for returning to the United States at the expiration of his current appointment on June 30, 1940, just six months ahead.

Chapter V

THE STORM GATHERS–
AND BREAKS

1940-1941

Mᴇᴀɴᴡʜɪʟᴇ it is essential to look at the political and military situation in which the College was operating. All of North China and the eastern seaboard had been under Japanese military occupation for more than two years. Almost every family in the PUMC, Chinese or foreign, was already separated by force of circumstances or facing such separation for an indefinite future; the cost of living was spiralling upwards; the occupying forces were tightening their control on every sector of life; censorship and surveillance were ever-present; friends and colleagues suddenly disappeared—one dared not inquire what had happened to them but the grapevine placed them in Japanese jails, held without charges or trial. What lay ahead? The implications of the widening war in the Western world were ominous. How long could the funds to support the College be safely remitted? The U.S. State Department renewed its pressures for the evacuation of women and children while sea routes were still open. Small wonder that there were frayed tempers, misunderstandings, criticisms, unreasonableness. The marvel is that in spite of all this there was so much real devotion to the institution and its purposes that students kept moving ahead in the regular progress of their medical and nursing training; patients filled the beds and clinics of the hospital to overflowing; research laboratories were active and productive, some 180 titles being published in 1938-39 and again in 1939-40. The arrival in early January

1940 of two visiting professors, Dr. Frank E. Burch in ophthalmology, and Dr. Irvine McQuarrie in pediatrics, each accompanied by his wife and Dr. McQuarrie with two teen-age daughters as well, gave a salutary sense of stability.

The cost of living continued to be of major concern and constant study. During the next six months this was discussed at practically every one of the nine meetings of the Business Division, leading to strong well-documented recommendations that won Trustee approval.

On February 21, 1940, Dr. Houghton told the Executive Committee that he would like to go to Chungking to attend a meeting of the North China Council for Rural Reconstruction of which the College had been a member since 1936. There he could explain the decision of the Trustees to withdraw the College as a participating member of this body, its removal from North China having made active cooperation impracticable at the present time. He also hoped to gather valuable information on medical activities in the interior and renew contacts with PUMC graduates and former staff. He doubted that this would create difficulties with the Japanese authorities in Peking since it was well known that the staff and students of the College had never been politically inclined. With the added assurance that work on the budget was already well under way and that he would be back in time for the Annual Meeting on March 27, the Executive Committee approved this "visit to the interior."

Most of the Trustees and staff agreed with Dr. Houghton's feeling that this trip could be made without harm to the College, but when they learned that he would be going in the company of President J. Leighton Stuart of Yenching University, many were apprehensive. Dr. Stuart was definitely a political figure, reputed to have close affiliations with the Nationalist Government in Chungking. They were fearful that no matter how discreet and nonpolitical Dr. Houghton might be, the Japanese would hold against him his association with Dr. Stuart on such a trip. Dr. Houghton was confident that this would not hurt the College, and events between his return and Pearl Harbor bore out that confidence.

Dr. Houghton was back in Shanghai as promised by March 27, 1940, for the Annual Meeting of the Trustees. As in December the five Shanghai Trustees together with Dr. Houghton constituted the quorum. This time Mr. Bowen was the financial officer present. Dr. Houghton reported on his recent trip, telling of the "splendid work" being done by PUMC graduates—medical and nursing—and former staff and graduate students. Most of the four-hour meeting was given over to financial matters—cost of living supplements and budget proposals for 1940-41. It was interesting to see how personal experience in the vagaries of exchange and rising commodity costs, the effect of military events on transportation and the concomitant skyrocketing of the price per ton of so vital a necessity as coal, affected Mr. Bowen's attitude toward the yardstick of the Stabilized Budget. As he came up against the harsh realities with which previous administrations had had to cope, they understandably irked him. He soon began to view stabilization as a desirable goal when external circumstances were in a state of "normalcy," but inapplicable in the face of the problems that beset the College as Japanese military control extended over a wider and wider area.

Mr. Bowen was therefore not perturbed that the 1940-41 budget totals showed no significant reduction from those for 1939-40 (including the supplementary appropriations made during the year). He pointed out to the Trustees how difficult it was under existing circumstances to make accurate estimates of what might be required in the way of subsistence allowances, and proposed that the Trustees ask the CMB to place at their disposal the total sum in US currency which was available for the year 1940-41, leaving it to the Trustees to apply this to the needs of the College at their discretion. This would obviate delays in adjusting subsistence allowances to sudden severe rises in living costs.

Mr. Bowen's suggestion found a sympathetic response from the Trustees as an opportunity to demonstrate that they really could be the independent and responsible custodians of the College's affairs the CMB and RF wished them to be. They accordingly asked the CMB for an appropriation of US$650,000 to cover the operation of the College according to the budget for 1940-41 and to leave a margin from which to cover such subsistence allowances and increased prices of materials and supplies as might be necessary.

The rest of this meeting was given over to routine business, but included one gratifying proposal—the appointment of Miss Vera Yu-chan Nieh as Dean of the School of Nursing to succeed Miss Gertrude E. Hodgman on September 15, 1940. Miss Nieh was herself a graduate of the School of which she would now be the first Chinese Dean.

With the election of new Trustees there were enough in North China to return the Executive Committee to the more convenient base of Peking. Dr. Houghton asked to be excused from re-election to the Board, reiterating his conviction that the Director should not serve on the Board. At the same time, the Trustees noted that his current appointment would expire on June 30, 1940, and asked the Governing Council for recommendations of candidates for Director. The long meeting ended with a special motion of appreciation for the work of the Acting Director, the other officers and the staff "in carrying on so efficiently under difficult circumstances, and for the support of the student body in this work."

Though gratified at this expression of genuine appreciation, Dr. Houghton again returned to Peking not at all certain that he would be interested in accepting reappointment should it be offered.

When the Governing Council met on April 17 and 18 to consider nominations for the post of Director, as requested by the Trustees, it was generally agreed that that post, which according to the Bylaws must be held by a Chinese, should in view of the current political situation, continue to remain vacant. A nominating committee of seven, representing the different sections of the institution, brought in a unanimous recommendation for the reappointment of Dr. Houghton as Vice Director, which was approved by the full membership of the Governing Council. The Executive Committee passed on this recommendation to the Chairman of the Board, Mr. Sohtsu G. King, who was in Shanghai, so that the official letter of appointment would have his endorsement.

Mr. King's letter offering appointment for a further period of three years from July 1, 1940, reached Peking early in May. Dr. Houghton did not reply immediately but by the middle of the month, after weighing all the factors involved, he wrote Mr. King accepting the appointment. His letter ended "I am grateful for your constant aid in the past and feel certain that I can count upon it during the uncertain and perhaps hazardous times that lie ahead of us all." These words were prophetic for in accepting this reappointment Dr. Houghton unknowingly was sentencing himself to four years as a prisoner of the Japanese Army.

Wartime Financing

The Trustees' request for a lump sum appropriation for the year 1940-41 had been sent to Mr. Lobenstine with a covering letter of explanation from Mr. King which ended with assurance of the PUMC Trustees' "loyal cooperation in adjusting our program accordingly" should the CMB's financial position make it necessary to provide a lesser amount. Mr. Lobenstine referred the budget and accompanying explanations to the Treasurer of The Rockefeller Foundation, Mr. E. R. Robinson, who on studying the figures questioned the validity of the rate of exchange used and expressed doubts as to the size of the margin proposed to cover possible increases in subsistence allowances and other unpredictable expenses, and cabled his questions and doubts to Peking. The reply of the Trustees answered his specific questions but ended with a renewed request for the wide contingency margin and a reminder that the Trustees needed early information as to what funds would be available for their discretionary use.

This message was brought in to the CMB Special Meeting held on Tuesday, May 21. That was the day—sometimes called Black Tuesday—when the German armies drove through the Allied lines in northern France toward the English channel. The New York papers carried accounts of widespread destruction in the areas of active fighting. The great Louvain Library, rebuilt after World War I , had again been completely destroyed. A German victory was recognized as a real possibility—but whatever the outcome, it was clear that the task of reconstruction of destroyed cities, towns and villages, of educational and other institutions would be tremendous.

Against this background, the members of the CMB trimmed the PUMC request for a lump sum grant of $650,000 to $480,000, broken down in designated blocks. Writing to Mr. King about this action, Mr. Lobenstine, after discussing the exchange rate, said that "it was felt that US$480,000 would provide both for the budgeted needs of the College and allow a sufficient sum to care for subsistence allowances." He remarked that "it was clearly realized that the much lower figure... would inevitably come as a shock to the Trustees and to the College administration" and "might be regarded as an expression of lack of confidence in the Trustees," but he asserted that this was not so. "If there is one thing more than another that characterizes the feeling in the China Medical Board, it is a growing conviction of the importance of strengthening the hands of the Trustees in every way possible. It is fully recognized here that the College is dependent for its successful functioning upon the continuance of a strong and influential Board of Trustees in China. The members of this Board are exceedingly thankful for those of you who are carrying heavy responsibilities on behalf of the College in China."

Interestingly enough, neither the Trustees nor Dr. Houghton took issue with this drastic reduction. Dr. Houghton wrote Mr. Lobenstine that the CMB actions had been "neither surprising nor particularly disappointing to any of us." There was a general realization of the situation created by world conditions, and readiness to "cheerfully accept the judgment of the Board... We will carry on to the best of our ability under the provisions made for our operation and, if no disastrous changes take place in local conditions, I feel sure that we can manage within the framework now provided."

Shortly after the May 21 meeting, the word reached New York that Dr. Houghton had accepted reappointment. Mr. Lobenstine had his own conception of how Dr. Houghton should handle his administrative responsibilities, a conception which he felt should now be clearly expressed to Dr. Houghton. He communicated his continued concern about this to Mr. Rockefeller, 3rd, with whom he was in frequent touch during the summer. Out of their discussions came the idea that a letter might be sent to Dr. Houghton advising him on the handling of his relationships with the Trustees and staff, while at the same time warning him that unlimited funds could not be counted on for the indefinite future.

Who should send such a letter? The choice was obvious—Mr. Rockefeller, Jr., whose warm personal relationship with Dr. Houghton went back to the very beginnings of the College, who had personally prevailed upon him to take on the delicate and thankless task of reorganization after the unhappy elimination of Mr. Greene, and who in 1938 had written him supporting the continuance of the tripartite RF-CMB-PUMC relationships and stressing the uncertainties of future financing. Once again Mr. Rockefeller was provided with copies of pertinent reports and correspondence and some drafted suggestions for the text, but the end result dated October 2, 1940, was unmistakably "Mr. Jr.'s" own.

While all this was under discussion in New York, the College was carrying on its normal pattern as far as this was possible. The Director's Annual Report for the year 1939-40 referred at the outset to the "momentous events" in recent months which might "gravely modify" the current program. The course of the war in Europe and in the Far East might well seriously affect such international undertakings as the PUMC. Dr.

Houghton reported that this "basic fact" was constantly in the minds of the officers who were devising contingent plans of action for the safety and welfare of the College. He pointed out that "under existing conditions it is impossible to see ahead; the circumstances of daily life—social, political, economic, military—alter with such rapidity that foresight is cancelled, and administrative measures exist for the needs of the moment only." It was not that there was any "immediate hazard, or that any specific dangers are now in sight; the essential issue is that our assurance of continuity is definitely less dependable than it was a half year ago."

The summer was spent, nevertheless, in preparing for an active school year. The first trimester opened in September 1940 with a total enrollment of 329 as against 281 the previous year, and 255 in 1938. While the entering classes were predominantly drawn from neighboring Yenching University, there were also students from Foochow, Canton, Shanghai, Soochow and Nanking, and even one venturesome American-born Chinese from the University of Illinois.

Everyone—staff and students alike—concentrated on maintaining as normal a program as possible. There were the usual parties and receptions for new students, and as the year went on the calendar showed regular meetings of the Faculty Medical Society, the Peking Section of the Society for Experimental Biology and Medicine, the Peking Society of Natural History and of less formal groups—one known as the Preclinical Tea, and another instituted by Dr. Houghton two or three years earlier called "Faculty Conversations"—which met monthly in the Director's living room for wide-ranging nonmedical discussions. The Department of Religious and Social Work which had been under the active fulltime leadership of the Rev. O. A. Griffiths since January 1940, maintained the Sunday morning services in the Auditorium and in addition encouraged a great variety of extracurricular activities.

One of the administrative changes for which the external situation was responsible was the recommendation by the Educational Division of the Governing Council that when the current appointment of Dr. C. E. Lim as Dean of the Medical School expired on June 30, 1940, that post should be held in abeyance for the time being, the Vice Director assuming the responsibilities of the Deanship until a more favorable atmosphere prevailed. Dr. Lim, chosen by his colleagues in 1937 and re-elected in the two succeeding years, had made an admirable dean. He had worked well with Dr. Houghton who, in line with the expressed policy of the Trustees and the CMB for "devolving responsibility upon the Chinese faculty and staff," had turned over to the Dean the Director's office in the main administration building, maintaining his own office in the Director's residence, the Ying Compound. The faculty had come to feel, however, that in a time of such uncertainty in the political environment it would be advantageous to the institution to centralize authority in one man, who should *not* be Chinese. With the Deanship vacant, on July 1 Dr. Houghton moved his office back to "C" Building, a step welcomed by the staff which found assurance in his accessibility and closer involvement in the many problems growing out of the increasing uncertainties of the external situation.

Mr. Rockefeller's letter reached Dr. Houghton about the middle of November. The letter which he had written two years earlier had been hung on the peg of the RF $2,000,000 pledge to the CMB to supplement its own income in support of the PUMC. The present letter came naturally out of remarks Mr. Rockefeller had made to The Rockefeller Foundation Trustees in April 1940 at the time of his retirement, in which he spoke at some length about the PUMC and the Foundation's further relationship to it. On that occasion he had expressed the hope that an additional and final gift of $5,000,000 would in due course be made to the CMB as an addition to the principal sums already in its hands available for carrying on the College. Referring to that statement in this letter to Dr. Houghton, he wrote that if the Board should vote this sum he would be "well pleased," that he thought it "highly improbable" that "under all the circumstances" it would vote more, but that he sincerely hoped it would not vote less.

He cautioned that even if this added principal fund should become available, readjustments, retrenchments, and even elimination of some services or departments would still be necessary. He quoted this surprising suggestion which he had made to the RF Trustees: "To operate on a self-supporting basis may be possible only by abandoning the Peking site and plant and, with a million or more of the endowment fund, building a far simpler plant, much less expensive to operate in the most strategic center of China." He was confident, however, that whatever steps must be taken it would be "without seriously impairing the usefulness of the institution or defeating the purpose for which it was established. In fact, such readjustments may be a blessing in disguise and in the long run only serve to strengthen the College and the better to insure its continued usefulness."

This led to what Mr. Lobenstine and Mr. Rockefeller, 3rd, felt was the heart of the matter, an emphasis less on money and more on "a whole-hearted spirit of cooperation between officers, trustees, faculty and students... All of these groups, as well as the Trustees of the Foundation and of the China Medical Board, are now looking to you to impart—as you so well can—that inspirational leadership, that spirit of unselfish subordination to the common good, of complete, wholehearted cooperation which is so greatly needed at this time. *With* such a spirit, its *present* funds will suffice to make the College a vital institution; *without* it, even were untold millions added, the College would never be worthy of its founders or its destiny."

Then recalling the fact that from the outset it had been contemplated that "within a reasonable period of time the institution should be taken over, maintained and operated by the Chinese, its Board, faculty and personnel having gradually become predominantly Chinese," he raised the question as to "whether the twenty years of existence which the College had rounded out does not constitute a 'reasonable period,' and whether the time is not fast approaching when responsibility for its future—both financial and medical—could and should be definitely assumed by the Chinese... Whether or not the actual moment for the transfer has come, the important thing is that such a transfer is both necessary and desirable and that no time should be lost in preparing the way for it."

The letter ended in Mr. Rockefeller's own warmly personal vein, assuring him of "our complete backing and our deep and abiding friendship." He recalled Dr. Houghton's rescue of Mrs. Rockefeller's sister, Miss Lucy Aldrich, many years before, when she had been kidnapped by bandits in Shantung Province, saying "I thank God that the immediate future of the Peking Union Medical College is in the hands of that courageous man. He did not fail us then, nor will he now."

Dr. Houghton received this letter in the spirit in which it was sent. All through the autumn his major efforts had been devoted to keeping the properties and program of the institution intact, to maintaining staff morale in the face of impending political changes and possible hardships, while quietly preparing plans of action to meet whatever turn local conditions might take. When Mr. Rockefeller's letter reached Peking in mid-November, the three Peking Trustees and his senior colleagues on the staff all agreed that it was desirable and at the moment feasible, for him to go to Shanghai to report on the state of the College to the seven Trustees (including the Chairman) who were there, and to discuss the implications of Mr. Rockefeller's letter. Dr. Houghton accordingly left Peking on November 26, returning on December 14 after numerous conferences. In an interim report he assured them that "the officers and staff will stand by, carrying on a full and active program as long as it is possible to do so," but cautioned that "the hold of the College upon continued existence is tenuous, because the supply and issue of coal is completely in the hands of the Japanese army" and if there should be any break in securing the College's minimum needs there would be "no alternative but to evacuate our patients in a few days and close the plant down. I speak of these possibilities not with any conviction that they will happen, but to acquaint you fully with the circumstances which face us, as the local course of war moves on to a crux."

On December 5, 1940, all the Trustees in Shanghai gathered for a meeting which had to be informal since they did not constitute a quorum. No official minutes were kept, but their reaction to Mr. Rockefeller's letter to Dr. Houghton was apparent from a letter to Mr. Rockefeller dated December 12, 1940, written by the Chairman, Mr. King. Unless it should become impossible to continue the College's program in Peking, the Trustees felt that a move to some other place would "cause misgiving and imply that the area is finished in China;" in addition they felt that "the transient situation in West China" was not "worthy of serious consideration for the establishment of permanent medical work." If major retrenchment should be necessary, the Trustees hoped that Dr. Gregg might first make a thorough survey of the situation on the spot, giving them his expert advice on how to proceed. As to possible changes in policy which might relate the College more closely to the national medical education program of China, the Trustees felt that "in the long run the high standards laid down provide the best possible leadership for the future medical work of the country." Mr. King stressed that "the Trustees are at one with you in recognizing that adequate emphasis on maintaining the spiritual life of the College is essential... recognizing that the pledges made must be maintained and for all time honorably kept." He went on

165

to say that "with regard to the creation of a greater spirit of loyalty and cooperation in the whole of the institution we... assure you of our wholehearted sympathy with and constant interest in promoting the welfare of the College, the individual work of its officers and staff and the morale of the student body." Mr. King then said the Trustees were "greatly honored that you should consider that it is desirable that a greater degree of responsibility should be transferred to us. Already we accept responsibility for the administration of the College and for the development and carrying out of its policies, and hope in due course that responsibility for its finance can be arranged."

The letter concluded with comments on the future financing of the College in the light of Mr. Rockefeller's suggestion for an additional gift of not less than $5,000,000 to the China Medical Board, saying first that the Trustees fully agreed that "whatever steps be taken, the usefulness of the institution must not be seriously impaired, nor the purposes for which it was established be defeated." Recalling Mr. Rockefeller's Dedication statement that one of the purposes was "to develop in China a medical school and hospital of a standard comparable with that of the leading institutions known to Western civilization" while keeping the cost of operation "on a conservative level," Mr. King wrote that "the Trustees fear that it will not be possible to maintain 'a wholly worth while medical college' within the limits of the proposed endowment." Again the hope was expressed that Dr. Gregg might be able to "come and help us evaluate the situation on the basis of China's needs."

Impact of World War II on Western Staff

Dr. Houghton also talked with the Shanghai Trustees at length on the question of evacuation of the families of American members of the staff in the light of the urgent advice being issued by the State Department and concurred in by the CMB. In November the wives and children of two American members of the faculty had left Peking to sail on the first of several special evacuation ships sponsored by the American authorities. There were other staff families who were uncertain what to do, and sought guidance from the administrative officers of the College. Out of the discussion of the Shanghai Trustees according to Dr. Houghton, "emerged a clear consensus of judgment that the Trustees should urge upon those concerned compliance with the suggestions of the State Department."

166

The group instructed Dr. Houghton to take the question up with the Executive Committee in Peking for "an official implementation of this decision." This he did immediately on his return, and on December 23, 1940, the Executive Committee took formal action "that foreign women and children (with the exception of women in staff positions the terms of whose appointments include specific insurance provision) be urged to leave China, with payment by the College of the travel expenses involved; that this action shall not be mandatory, individual family units being free to make their own decisions in the light of their particular circumstances; that staff families who decide to remain in China shall communicate this decision and the reasons therefor to the Trustees through the Acting Director, together with an assumption of their full responsibility in any eventuality." The action included families of the few non-American Western members of the staff who were also likely to be affected by any grave change in the local situation.

In the two months immediately after this, five "family units" left under these provisions; six others decided to stay together in Peking, in each case signing a statement of "full responsibility for deciding to remain in China at this time" and freeing the Trustees and officers of the College "from all obligation arising from this decision." As the winter wore on, the list of wives and children leaving on one or another of the "President" liners—the Coolidge, Pierce, Taft—lengthened and the men who stayed behind shared bachelor quarters or moved in with some remaining family.

On March 26, 1941, Dr. Houghton was once again in Shanghai, this time for the Adjourned Annual (1941) Meeting which nine Trustees succeeded in attending, an actual majority of the whole Board—the largest attendance at such a meeting since March 27, 1937. The formal business followed the normal pattern. No controversial items were on the docket; the budget formulated in US$ and LC$ showed no important change from that for the previous year, and it was left to the CMB to determine the exchange rate at which the covering US$ appropriation should be reckoned. It is interesting to note that when the CMB acted on this request two months later, they came up with an overall total of US$510,500—$30,500 more than the total for the previous year.

For many of the Trustees this Annual Meeting was their first chance in several years to talk with each other and with Dr. Houghton, and the meeting lasted for more than five hours, most of which was devoted to

167

off-the-record discussion of the future of the College in terms of existing political and military developments. Dr. Houghton's interim report covering the period since July 1, 1940, formed the basis for this exchange of views. Starting out with the comment that it is probably fortunate that one cannot always see clearly into the future "for courage might falter at the vision," he said that "the year thus far has been lived from day to day, with an eye to needs and tasks immediately at hand and with no effort at prophecy." In spite of this, "from the angle of achieving the basic aims of the College, the academic year 1940-41 has probably been the most successful year in the history of the institution... The number of students (graduate and undergraduate, in medicine and nursing) is as large as it ever was; in the hospital our greatest problem is not a lack of material, but the crowding of patients applying for care beyond the capacity of the plant and the time and strength of the professional personnel. The narrowing of social outlets and diversions has resulted in an increased amount of time spent in researches and investigations of various sorts... The net result of environmental conditions has been... a year of intense activity in the College, and a corresponding sense of satisfaction and achievement on the part of those concerned. Continuity of our program is still gravely uncertain... one may not forget that what has thus far been a scene of continental conflict now becomes only a small corner in the arena of world war and necessarily shares in the ebb and flow of events far removed from this place... We can only keep a cheery hope that somehow a way will be found to keep going in the future as in the past, and to meet the urgent demands that have been laid upon the College and its Hospital." Returning to Peking, Dr. Houghton was heartened by a warm sense of Trustee backing and understanding of the complexity and unpredictability of the problems which the College administration had to face.

Mr. V. F. Bradfield, Treasurer of the College, resigned at this time. Mr. Bowen's original appointment as Controller in 1935 had been on a short-term basis, but the Trustees had continued his appointment so that there would be two financial officers, one of whom would devote himself primarily to the anticipated investment program. But such a program was not immediately forthcoming, and Mr. Bowen had gradually absorbed more and more of the functions once carried by the Treasurer alone. Mr. Bradfield agreed with the Trustees that without an investment program there was no need for two senior financial officers so that he felt justified in asking to be relieved of his duties in order to return to the United States to care more adequately for his heavy family responsibilities. His resignation was accepted by the Executive Committee on April 23, 1941, "with unqualified regret." His service had been long and valuable and he would be greatly missed. Before leaving he had prepared detailed inventories of the whole institution which he took to the China Medical Board at Dr. Houghton's request. No one then foresaw how important these would prove to be in substantiating the eventual claim for war losses filed by the China Medical Board with the U.S. War Claims Commission, which in 1967 resulted in a payment to the CMB of more than $1,200,000.

The frequent letters from Dr. Houghton throughout the summer and autumn give a vivid picture of how the College was affected by the rapidly deteriorating war situation. Dr. Houghton had "small hope" if war should eventuate, that there would be any way for the College to continue its work. Operation under the direction of a neutral with funds supplied from New York? This was dubious, but it might be worth trying. "Failing that, the staff would have to be liquidated and the plant either sealed or confiscated." It would probably be necessary not only to evacuate the remaining women but also to send with them any of the American men who wished to go while there was a chance of getting out. He and Mr. Bowen had no thought of leaving. Dr. Houghton was trying to avoid needless stirring up of anxiety and rumor. "You will realize how easily fantastic stories and whisperings run around a small community like ours and how readily people under emotional tension surrender their common sense." The ordinary program of the College would be continued until and unless forcibly interrupted. Appointments and reappointments of a large number of graduate students, fellows, externes and demonstrators for the coming year had been routinely offered, and all had been accepted. Between fifty and sixty applications for admission to the first year of medical studies had been filed, with more in prospect—a much larger group than ever before. A large entering class in nursing was also expected. All preparations were for a normal year.

At the end of May the school year was drawing to a successful close with final examinations and Commencement scheduled as usual. Customary entrance examinations in various centers were being planned for, and routine preparations for the next academic session were under way.

Preparing for Emergencies

On May 24, 1941, the Executive Committee empowered the Chairman and Acting Director in an emergency to take such steps as might be required to safeguard the personnel and property of the College—this was to cover any sudden need for action when there was no time to call the Executive Committee together. With the possibility of a situation calling for immediate liquidation, the CMB was asked to put a three months' reserve of operating funds in the hands of the College officers as of July 1, against which it would be possible to draw in case the transmission of money between Peking and the United States should be interrupted. "The amount required for complete liquidation of Chinese staff and employees would be approximately FRB$2,000,000." (FRB was the designation of the new local currency).

Pressure on the outpatient clinics and wards of the Hospital was so heavy that it was necessary to devise some practical way in which to lessen the load. Patients referred elsewhere preferred to wait almost indefinitely for an appointment at the PUMC. "It may be flattering, but it is also embarrassing us, and unsafe for the patient."

The Trustees were still eager to have Dr. Gregg visit the College and on May 24, 1941, the Executive Committee requested the CMB to arrange this for the purpose of aiding the Trustees and officers to survey the College in connection with the proposals for a new financial basis of operation. Everyone realized that the political and military situation might not be favorable, but hope continued that Dr. Gregg might be able to go to Peking in the early autumn for two or three months.

By the end of June the recent outbreak of German-Soviet hostilities was a new factor in the political and military possibilities in the Pacific area. Most of the President liners were being withdrawn from trans-Pacific service, and all reservations after early July had been cancelled. If other sailings should materialize it might yet be possible to get the fellows on their way to the United States in the near future, as well as faculty members wishing to leave. At the same time, graduates and Chinese staff members who wished to go to the "interior" were finding increasing difficulties in financing the cost of travel for their families and themselves, and Dr. Houghton suggested that some assistance might be given them on their arrival through grants from The Rockefeller Foundation Division of Medical Education.

A month later Dr. Houghton wrote that financial help to those wanting to go to West China was "now probably only an academic question" since new regulations were being enforced which would make it very difficult for "our Chinese" to leave Peking. Recent shifting of Japanese troops into Manchuria had caused great deterioration in train service out of Peking. Only eight trains were still running. No steamers to Kobe or Dairen were available and no "foreigners (except Chinese)" were allowed to enter Japan. And yet "within the College all routines are now going on as usual." Entrance examinations for the Medical School were over and a large entering class was expected in the autumn. In the School of Nursing twenty of the entering class had reported for the summer session. The Hospital was still too crowded. Coal stocks were being maintained at a level of approximately eight thousand tons, and deliveries were regular. Supplies of staple foods had been built up to a six months' reserve.

These reports and other correspondence went regularly from Peking but their arrival in New York was unpredictable, sometimes taking as long as three months on the way. They were of necessity supplemented by telegraphic and radio communications, sometimes through State Department and American Embassy channels when it was important to avoid the eyes of the censor, and again through open channels which were usually quicker. Of special concern both in New York and in Peking was how to assure adequate bank balances in Peking to meet emergencies with minimum danger of loss of any substantial sum through freezing measures or outright confiscation. The CMB Finance Committee in response to the request for a three months' reserve of operating funds, took the conservative course of providing two weeks' requirements on the assumption that should the United States freeze such accounts it would not take more than two weeks to secure a license.

When the U.S. Treasury Department on July 26, 1941, did freeze all accounts of individuals and organizations in the Far East subject to Treasury licenses for each transaction, the full implications of this action were not at first understood by Mr. Bowen who continued to pay bills and draw on New York accounts as usual. This brought him a warning from Mr. Robinson in New York against using any funds of the College "in any manner to contravene the regulations of the Treasury Department." Mr. Bowen on his part rather enjoyed finding paths through and around difficulties which might have blocked someone less adventurous,

171

reporting to Mr. Robinson that he was working closely with the local branch of the National City Bank "devising ways and means for continuing to do business in spite of the regulations... we are one of the few enterprises still doing business... we are continuing to do a little honest business only by circumlocutory methods. If these business regulations do not yield at one point we try another. I realize also of course that our occasional resort to panzer movements would not get far with your 'regulations.' However I promise to be good, and to keep at least one eye on the traffic lights."

The summer and autumn of 1941 were very frustrating months for the members of the CMB and for Mr. Lobenstine in particular—everyone urgently looking for ways to protect the College and its staff and somehow to conserve as much as possible for the future, but powerless to do much more than attempt to keep the pipelines of support open. Between May 21 and November 17 there were no formal meetings of the CMB, but there were frequent informal consultations in New York and Washington. Mr. Lobenstine corresponded at length with all the members, passing on to them whatever news came from Dr. Houghton, or from his many missionary and governmental contacts.

In one of Mr. Lobenstine's cables to Dr. Houghton, he said that the CMB would "view with favor" some arrangement to conserve the medical faculty by temporary allocation of personnel to medical institutions in West China, the CMB paying necessary transportation and maintenance costs. After replying by cable that the "entire program" was going on "normally" and there was "no occasion for alarm," Dr. Houghton commented by letter that he was glad to have this word. This was something the Trustees had been considering from various angles during the past year, but it had not been practicable to make fixed and definite plans or to discuss the subject openly, for it was necessary to bear in mind constantly "that this area is under military occupation, tightening from month to month as war and economic conditions worsen." It was not possible to say whether or not any considerable number of the faculty could get out safely. "Certainly no general movement could be undertaken, and whatever is to be prepared for, or done, must be arranged with the utmost discretion. The College itself cannot appear as a party to such a scheme, for the military high command would deal with us instantly under such conditions. On the other hand, there are definite steps that may be taken, now that we have an indication that the Board will assist in carrying out some such plan... I am endeavoring to make a prompt contact with the Shanghai Trustees for their help would be a major item." Dr. Houghton succeeded in getting down to Shanghai by sea from the port of Ching-wantao, and on August 25, 1941, met informally with the Shanghai Trustees to discuss the general situation and in particular the CMB's interest in the transferring of the faculty to West China.

Their conclusions as reported to Mr. Lobenstine by Dr. Houghton were: (1) that the Japanese would be against continuation even of such "non-political humanitarian public service" as hospital work, the strong probability being that the Japanese army would utilize the plant or would force the local government to use it, with Japanese doctors in key positions. Consent to continue operation would imply arranging to receive the necessary funds through a neutral legation with a neutral national in nominal control, Dr. Hoeppli, a Swiss citizen, being the only present member of the staff who would qualify. (2) "It is out of the question to contemplate transferring the College to another place, or even to shift faculty members in any considerable numbers." The journey west, "long, rough, hazardous" could only be done "furtively" and only by men — which would mean families staying behind for whom financial provisions would have to be made. (3) The sudden closing of the College in order to move the faculty gradually to the west, would be a "difficult and delicate task" requiring several weeks. It would make a great stir locally, every important staff member would be a marked man, and none could be moved quietly away.

The course of choice therefore appeared to the Trustees to be continuance of the program as at present, in the hope that open warfare might not eventuate, and in the meantime to make ready as far as possible for whatever particular circumstance might arise. If war should come, and some of the faculty should succeed in reaching West China, there would be no problem attaching them to one or another of the medical schools or research institutions already there, or in continuing payment of their salaries. Dr. Wong Wen-hao, the senior Trustee in Chungking, was being asked by the Chairman of the Board to organize a special committee of Trustees in West China to take charge on behalf of the Board of Trustees of whatever arrangements might need to be made, and to communicate with the officers in New York.

In the meantime, cables were going back and forth through regular channels about arrangements to be made for Chinese fellows in the United States who were having trouble in getting passage back to China, about deposits for wives who were finding it difficult to clear frozen bank accounts, about State Department visas for individuals already en route to the United States. One such cable dated October 16 ended "All quiet here."

On October 9 a cable from New York gave Dr. Houghton the regretted—though not unanticipated—word that Dr. Gregg's visit had been indefinitely postponed owing to the impossibility of any long-range planning under existing circumstances. It included a message from Mr. Fosdick assuring Dr. Houghton that the interest of the College would not suffer by the delay in securing Dr. Gregg's advice.

The Executive Committee of the Trustees met on November 12 in Peking, following which Mr. Ballou, its chairman, sent a cable to Mr. Lobenstine through the State Department reporting that it was anticipated that "in case the conversations in Washington do not satisfy the desires of those in control here," it was expected that American institutions at Peking would be closed by withdrawing permits to transact business or purchase supplies. "In such an eventuality," the PUMC could not continue to operate and the Trustees would seal the institution and liquidate the contracts of all of the staff and employees. To do this the PUMC would need to have in cash in Peking FRB$1,750,000, a sum which would have to be built up gradually in order to prevent exchange going against the College. The Executive Committee asked the CMB to deposit US$175,000 with the National City Bank of New York subject to draft by the Tientsin office of the bank. The local currency obtained would be used for liquidation, if necessary, or if not required for that purpose would remain on deposit in local currency "under appropriate safeguards." Meanwhile the usual monthly deposits of the CMB would cover current operating expenses. In addition about $250,000 would be required in New York for travel and liquidation of the foreign staff. The cable ended with assurance of the determination of the Trustees "to carry on as long as possible a normal program."

All these financial arrangements were off-the-record as far as the Minutes of the meeting of the Executive Committee on November 12 are concerned, but the Minutes record a statement of general principles, covering

174

the contractual obligations of the College applicable to members of the staff under differing circumstances. These forward-looking statements which did not reach New York until March 10, 1942, were invaluable to the CMB during the war years in handling the cases of those staff members who were in the United States and those who reached West China.

The final action of the Executive Committee on November 12 was a statement adopted for circulation among the staff and students who were disturbed by rumors that the College was about to close:

To All Staff Members and Students:

The Trustees view with satisfaction the way in which the College and Hospital have maintained their manifold activities during the recent year. It is their desire and expectation that this normal state of affairs will continue. No change in the program of the College will be contemplated unless necessitated by circumstances beyond the control of the Trustees. The loyal cooperation of staff and students in carrying on their work as usual is asked.

Less than a month later, those "circumstances beyond the control of the Trustees" took place at Pearl Harbor, and in the Philippines.[*]

Mr. Ballou's cable was received the day after a Special Emergency Meeting of the CMB to discuss new regulations of the Stabilization Board in Washington which would seriously affect the exchange rate and the cost of meeting the College budget. The discussion took place in the light of "the fact that war with Japan appeared imminent" to quote the CMB minutes, and covered CMB responsibility to the remaining foreigners on the staff, possible continuance of the PUMC under a neutral head, and the necessity of revising the budget in terms of the "new conditions." On November 21 the Executive Committee met again to review the situation in the light of Mr. Ballou's message, and after further discussion approved a reply to Mr. Ballou to be sent through the State Department stating that government regulations would delay the transmission of funds, asking what local and American funds the College had on hand, stating that the CMB did not anticipate an immediate break, asking to be kept informed of any changes in plans or in the local situation, and ending with a statement that the Trustees and Dr. Houghton had the "fullest confidence" of the CMB.

On November 26 a reply to this message was received by commercial radiogram saying that there was no money on hand, the November remit-

---

[*] In the Western world the attack on Pearl Harbor was made on December 7, 1941; for those in the Eastern hemisphere it fell on December 8th.

tance was being awaited, Mr. Ballou had left Peking, and ending with the familiar "all quiet here." The day the cable was received in New York, Mr. Robinson remitted US$40,000.

During the next ten days, Mr. Lobenstine and the members of the CMB were in almost continuous telephone contact with each other and with the State Department. By December when the prospects of a peaceful outcome to the Japanese-American negotiations seemed more unlikely than ever, they had concluded that they must be prepared to make available the full $175,000 Mr. Ballou's cable had asked for. On November 29 the sum of US$180,000 was remitted through the Chase Bank through its Shanghai and Hong Kong branches, and a message through the State Department was sent to Dr. Houghton reporting this, ending with the gloomy statement that there was no indication that the American government would alter its "present stand," and the warning that "foreigners deciding to remain need to be prepared for all eventualities." A cable received from Dr. Houghton on December 1 said "while situation here is getting worse, things are quiet."

The College *Weekly Bulletin* for December 3, 1941, listed on its Calendar "Monday, December 8. Regular Instruction of Second Trimester Begins" and gave a preliminary summary of the College plans for the Christmas season—the usual Christmas Greetings Club, the College party, carol singing in the hospital wards on Christmas Eve. It was six years before this familiar news sheet was published again.

On December 6 a commercial cable about the plans of one of the fellows in the United States signed by the head of his department, Dr. Loucks, as well as by Dr. Houghton, included the statement "we anticipate college will continue normally."

On Sunday, December 7, everyone who had access to a short-wave radio sat up late listening to President Roosevelt's appeal to the Japanese Emperor for restraint of the Japanese military.

The next morning, Monday, December 8, 1941, the storm struck. Shortly before eight o'clock a detachment of Japanese soldiers entered the PUMC Hospital, closed all gates and threw a cordon around the premises so that no one could go in or out. Simultaneously soldiers went to the Director's residence at Ying Compound where Dr. Houghton was at breakfast with Mr. Bowen and Dr. Anderson whose families had left. Dr. Loucks, who had spent several hours with Dr. Houghton the previous evening discussing steps to be taken in case of a final break between Japan and the United

States, heard of Pearl Harbor on the 8:00 a. m. radio broadcast from Shanghai and rushed to the telephone to reach Dr. Houghton. Mr. Bowen replied "Yes, we have learned the news. Japanese soldiers are now coming through our front door."

Dr. Houghton and Mr. Bowen were taken into custody forthwith. Four long years as prisoners of the Japanese army lay ahead of them.

Chapter VI

PEARL HARBOR
AND THE WAR YEARS

1941-1945

THE BURDEN of meeting the immediate situation, when the Japanese soldiers entered and cordoned off the Hospital on the morning of December 8, 1941 fell on the nursing service and resident doctors. They remained calmly at their regular work, thus keeping the patients from apprehension.

December 8 happened to be the first day of the scheduled examination of the senior nursing students by the Nurses Association of China. Miss Nieh, Dean of the School of Nursing, and Miss Faye Whiteside, Superintendent of Nurses, had come on duty before eight to greet the two examiners sent by the NAC, who fortunately arrived just before the Japanese closed the gates. Later Miss Nieh reported to the Trustees that with all entrances guarded by Japanese soldiers it was obvious that "something serious must have happened" but it was several hours before anyone knew just what the situation was. In the meantime, the nurses already on the wards went about their usual routines and the NAC examinations went on undisturbed. The students were told that Japanese soldiers were visiting the hospital (a not unusual occurrence) so when any of the occupying troops looked into the classroom, the girls paid them no heed but kept at their examination papers. These examinations continued for the usual three days, so that circumstances notwithstanding, members of the nursing Class of 1942 were duly qualified by the Nurses Association of China, an essential for government registration after graduation. This incident was characteristic of the imperturbability with which the whole student body and staff throughout the institution met the crisis.

By Tuesday, most members of the staff, including "enemy aliens," were permitted to report for duty—even urged by the military to do so. Within a week all were at work as usual and the officer in command gave permission for students to come to classes and regular class work was resumed on December 15. In the Hospital, however, by order of the commanding officer no new patients were admitted to the wards after December 8 and the outpatient clinics were closed from that date on. Patients already in the Hospital were allowed to stay on, but future operation did not look promising.

The commanding officer took possession of the keys to the institution and set up his office in that of Dr. S. T. Wang, the Superintendent of the Hospital. Dr. Houghton and Mr. Bowen were taken to the barracks of the U.S. Marines where they were held for the next month with a mixed group of other enemy aliens, out of touch with friends and colleagues, all speculating uneasily about the future. On January 8, all of their companions were released, without questioning, and sent home on parole, with the exception of Dr. I. Snapper, the Dutch Professor of Medicine at the PUMC, and President J. L. Stuart of Yenching University, who together with Dr. Houghton and Mr. Bowen were taken to Ying Compound, still prisoners under guard. The comfort of Dr. Houghton's home was a welcome relief after the rigors of the previous month, but they were still sequestered, and very uncertain about the future.

On January 19, the Superintendent, Dr. S. T. Wang, and the only senior administrative officer still functioning, was notified by the commanding officer that classes must be discontinued that day, that the preclinical departments should be closed by the end of the week, and that all students must leave the main buildings within two days—staying in the dormitories only until arrangements for departure could be made. The various women's dormitories, medical and nursing, were closed on January 31; the men's dormitory closed on February 7.

Each undergraduate student before leaving was given a transcript of his record in the Medical School or School of Nursing. The Educational Division of the Governing Council held an extraordinary meeting on January 19 at which the members of the two senior classes, medical and nursing, were granted degrees and diplomas normally due in June. No graduation exercises were held but the graduates were given makeshift diplomas signed by Dr. Houghton—an appreciated act of leniency from the commanding officer—and were able to have a class picture taken in the distinctive PUMC cap and gown.

Up until January 19 when the order came to disband the students, hope had been entertained that it might be possible to continue operation of the College or at least of the Hospital, under reduced budget and local control. A group of senior Chinese members of the staff had labored diligently to prepare plans and secure support for such a measure.

Dr. Wang's first step on January 19 was to call together the senior staff of the whole institution to discuss the Hospital's future. The house staff, like the students, would soon be dispersed. There were still some 130 patients in the Hospital whom the commanding officer was willing to have remain as long as necessary with such medical and nursing staff as was needed for their care, but no new patients would be admitted for the duration of the war. After full discussion there was unanimous agreement that it would be best for all concerned to close the whole institution, discharging or transferring all patients from the Hospital before that date. The last patients were discharged on January 28, and on Saturday, January 31, the staff was paid, cash on hand making it possible to give one month's additional salary to all Chinese employees. As each one received his pay, he turned in his identification pass and left the buildings, carrying his personal property with him (a privilege also given to students). The PUMC was now completely in the hands of the Japanese.

The War Years—Peking

For a large number of people in Peking, February 1, 1942, marked the beginning of an uncertain future. The PUMC had been the axis around which their lives revolved and on which their families depended for their daily living, while for students it was the foundation of their professional lives. What to do now?

Continued attempts to transfer to some other hospital a large Chinese unit including senior staff, juniors, house staff, nurses and technical personal, were fruitless—the Japanese did not favor the idea of continuing the PUMC tradition elsewhere. (In spite of this many were taken on the staff of the Chung Ho (Central) Hospital one by one, so that in the course of a year or so they constituted a real PUMC group). Some found oppor-

180

tunities to slip through the lines to the West, but when families were involved this was sufficiently hazardous to deter many who otherwise would have gone. Many of the senior staff, after helping recent graduates to place themselves, went into private practice in Peking or in Tientsin. Some of the younger ones set up group practice.

The lowest paid employee group turned to various ways of making a living—working as day laborers, peddling peanuts and fruit, pulling rickshaws or operating the new three-wheelers—but times were very hard for many. It was the clerical staff who were the hardest hit for their chief tool, familiarity with the English language, had become a handicap and openings were few.

Many students went to their homes in the Shanghai area. Medical students were taken in by St. John's and the National Medical College of Shanghai. Nursing students were absorbed into various hospitals. In the north, medical students were accepted by the Medical College of the National University. Miss Nieh arranged for the first and second year nursing students to transfer to the Nurses Training School of the Presbyterian Douw Hospital, and for senior students to complete their practical experience in hospitals in Peking and Tientsin.

The members of the Board of Trustees were scattered to Tientsin, Shanghai, West China and the United States. Only three were in Peking, one serving his first term and so physically handicapped that he could not leave his house. It was obviously impossible and probably unwise to try to hold the usual Annual Meeting of the Board anywhere, but several trustees met informally in Shanghai in April 1942, sharing what information had filtered down from the north about the closing of the institution. They were anxious to maintain some thread of organization to facilitate as far as possible the handling of any matters requiring official attention. In view of the continuing isolation of Dr. Houghton, they asked Dr. Loucks whose movements around Peking were not seriously restricted, to serve temporarily as Acting Director, with a supporting committee consisting of Dr. S. T. Wang, Mr. James S. Ch'en, and Miss Mary E. Ferguson, to represent the Hospital, the business administration, and the general administration. In the eyes of the local authorities, the PUMC was of course defunct, but this group kept in frequent touch to discuss the general situation and interests of the College. When the opportunity came to send a report to other members of the Board of Trustees and to the

China Medical Board, Inc., by hand of American diplomatic representatives being repatriated on the first Japanese-American exchange in May 1942, this group together with the two accessible trustees, Dr. S. D. Wilson and Mr. T. A. Sun, sent a detailed account of events since Pearl Harbor. When their report reached New York it was the first comprehensive news of all that had happened in the past six months—very welcome to all who were concerned about relatives and friends but discouraging to those who had kept hope that somehow as a humanitarian institution the PUMC might still continue to carry on some service.

Meanwhile Dr. Houghton and Mr. Bowen had been moved on May 8, 1942, together with President Stuart and Dr. Snapper, from the relatively comfortable existence at Ying Compound to 45 Wai Chiao Pu Chieh, the commandeered residence and offices of an English businessman. From that date no visitors were allowed at all, and their isolation was absolute until August 1945, except for occasional censored letters and the local Japanese-run English language daily newspaper. Their constant hope was for repatriation on one of the prospective exchanges of Japanese and Allied civilians. Dr. Snapper and his wife, who had joined him in detention at Ying Compound, were allowed at the last moment to leave on one of these exchanges in August 1942, but the remaining trio were not so fortunate.

Before Pearl Harbor, many had assumed that when the anticipated blow fell, there would be a general internment and even had suitcases of basic necessities ready in case of a sudden move. These apprehensions did not immediately materialize. It was not until March 12, 1943, that instructions for general internment in a former Presbyterian Mission school compound at Weihsien, Shantung, were finally issued. All the remaining "enemy aliens" on the PUMC staff were sent there with two exceptions— the British chief engineer who was kept to supervise the power plant in the walled British Embassy Compound where persons exempted for reasons of health or age were sent, and an American woman who was allowed to remain with her ailing father.

In September 1943, the long-delayed Second American Exchange finally took place, bringing back to New York on December 1, 1943, all PUMC Americans except for the Chinese-Americans whom the Japanese did not consider American citizens, a few others who chose to stay with friends in the Weihsien camp, and the hapless Dr. Houghton and Mr. Bowen. Their names had actually been on the approved list for this exchange, but were removed by the local Japanese high command without explanation. Not even the Swiss authorities representing American interests were able to get permission to visit them, nor did the strongest pressure by the U.S. State Department and every possible influential source, succeed in securing their release and repatriation.

For the prisoners of war in Peking the future stretched out in what Dr. Houghton described in his journal as "an infinity of bleak silence." Temperatures in their cramped quarters varied between 8° in mid-winter to near 110° in summer. Although Mr. Bowen on one occasion went through several far from pleasant days of intensive questioning as to the whereabouts of the "Peking Man" skull, and other important anthropological materials, and Dr. Stuart was subjected to periodic and prolonged interrogations, they were never told why they had been arrested, no formal charges were ever made nor were they ever tried and sentenced. It was a test of physical and psychological endurance. The first ray of hope was sight of the first American plane over Peking, recorded in Dr. Houghton's diary on January 25, 1945. Ten days later another plane was seen. On May 6 news reached them of German capitulation—hope grew stronger. On July 24, Dr. Houghton recorded "a bolt from a clear sky"—a visit to Dr. Stuart by his personal secretary, Mr. Philip Fugh, accompanied by a Japanese Colonel. Several other visits were made by Mr. Fugh, who on August 11, assured them that Japan had agreed to the Allies' terms and the end was only a matter of days. On August 15, he brought word that the war was really over, the Japanese had surrendered, and capitulation would be signed the next day.

Unfortunately for the eager trio, local conditions in Peking delayed their immediate release. It was a question of whether the Japanese would surrender to the Communist 8th Route Army just outside the city walls, or wait for Nationalist troops to appear. There was great confusion. Even the Swiss Consul and other friends, armed with permits from the Gendarmerie, found their permits countermanded by some Japanese bureaucrat. Finally on August 17, Dr. Hoeppli arrived with a Japanese consular officer to take the three men "at once" to Gendarmerie Headquarters for their formal release. This called for a speech by the Commandant, handshaking, exchange of bows—the long ordeal was incredibly over.

A few days of greatly needed rest and relaxation, one quick visit to the

PUMC, which was far from its former spotless self and was still full of Japanese, and Dr. Houghton was flown by American Army plane to the southwest on the first leg of his journey to New York where he arrived on September 11. Home at last.

Mr. Bowen had chosen to stay on in Peking, holding a letter from Dr. Houghton authorizing him to receive the plant from the Japanese on behalf of the owners whenever it should be rendered. Dr. Stuart and Philip Fugh had flown to Chungking for consultation with Yenching colleagues.

On September 27, 1945, Dr. Houghton made a brief report to the Trustees at a Special Meeting called to welcome his safe return and to discuss first steps in planning for the future of the College. Reporting on the cursory view he had had before leaving Peking the end of August, Dr. Houghton said that structurally the buildings seemed undamaged, but the whole property was filthy, much of the movable or removable equipment seemed to be gone, the power plant appeared to need complete replacement before any extensive load could be put upon it. Obviously rehabilitation of the physical plant was to be a major undertaking for the future administration. The brightest spot in the picture was the fact that the library and clinical records appeared to be intact, the Japanese having left these in charge of the College Librarian, Mr. T. F. Chao, under the protective supervision of a Japanese conscript doctor, Major Matsuhashi, who in pre-war days had himself used the PUMC library and appreciated its scientific importance.

Some twenty-four years later in an assessment of total losses incurred by the CMB when the institution was taken over by the Peoples Republic of China, the Library was valued at not less than US$2,000,000. Its real value, however, could never be expressed in monetary terms. Made up as it was of the outstanding collections of books, pamphlets, and complete sets of journals which the CMB had the foresight to purchase for the College in Germany at the end of World War I , added to year by year under the wise supervision of the faculty's Committee on the Library, and including the remarkable collection of Chinese books[*] on the classical system of medicine acquired in 1936-37, it was properly described in one report as constituting "the most valuable intellectual endowment of the College." Beginning with the year 1925 the chairmanship of the Library Committee

---

[*] Fortunately not long before Pearl Harbor, microfilm copies of this collection were sent to the United States. These are now in the custody of the Library of Congress.

alternated between Dr. Chester N. Frazier and Dr. R. Hoeppli, two men from whose devotion to the maintenance of the Library at a high level of excellence the College, faculty and students, received incalculable benefits.

The War Years — New York

With the actual outbreak of war, the first concern of the CMB was what might have happened to the personnel and the property of the PUMC. During the first frantic week after Pearl Harbor inquiries went by cable directly to Chinese trustees in Chungking, and through the Swiss Minister in Washington to Swiss officials in Shanghai and Peking. It was December 31 when the first word was received in New York — sent by the Swiss Consul General in Shanghai to the Swiss Minister in Washington who telephoned the brief message to Mr. Fosdick at the Rockefeller Foundation offices in New York: *College and Hospital continue to function. Staff all well.* (signed) *Loucks.* This was of course good news, but why was it signed by Dr. Loucks? What had happened to Dr. Houghton? Two weeks later the Swiss Minister again reported a cable, this time from Dr. Hoeppli, whose Swiss citizenship and official service representing the Shanghai Swiss Consul General in charge of American interests were to stand the institution in such good stead throughout the war, repeating the substance of the first cable, but still no mention of Dr. Houghton. It was not until early February that Dr. Houghton was permitted by the Japanese to ask Dr. Hoeppli to send a message through Swiss channels, a message which reached New York a whole month later, conveying the information that the PUMC had been discontinued on February 1 by order of the military; that he, Mr. Bowen and Dr. Snapper were "held in custody but well treated and in good health;" asking that they be included in any exchange of non-resident aliens which might prove "feasible."

This direct word was of course a welcome relief to the anxiety about Dr. Houghton's fate. From then on, as exchange negotiations with Japan were undertaken by the allied governments, the Board unremittingly pressed for the repatriation of all "enemy nationals" on the staff with special emphasis on the release of Dr. Houghton, Mr. Bowen, and Dr. and Mrs. Snapper, efforts eventually effective for all except Dr. Houghton and Mr. Bowen.

Early attention was given to the question of various payments which the CMB had been accustomed to make at the request of the College and as a convenience to individual staff members. These included salary and other payments to staff members and families who were outside China on leave of absence or fellowships. In addition there were now those caught in Manila at the outbreak of war on their way home; still others were families of staff members, who had previously returned in response to State Department urgings while their husbands and fathers stayed in Peking. At a Special Meeting of the CMB on December 18, 1941, less than two weeks after Pearl Harbor, an emergency appropriation was approved "for use in making payments ordinarily charged to appropriations made directly to the PUMC" subject to reassuring provisions which made it clear that no one was going to be left high and dry.

Aside from the small number of Chinese staff members in the United States covered by these provisions, the Board was deeply concerned about the condition of the large number of Chinese, professional and non-professional, in Peking whose livelihood had been so abruptly cut off. Unfortunately there was no possibility of further remittances to North China. For the time being, all that could be done was to keep their annuity policies active and to seek ways of helping individuals who might make their way to southwest China.

One other important decision of the CMB at that time was to maintain subscriptions to scientific periodicals for the College Library, so that when the war was over the file of journals in Peking would be unbroken. All through the war years the CMB never lost confidence that some day the College would be reopened.

While thus protecting the present and future needs of the PUMC, its staff and students, there was a strong feeling in the CMB that the Board should make some direct contribution to the general medical needs of Free China through grants for such purposes—salaries, student aid, teaching supplies and emergency building needs. The Board turned first to Dr. Marshall C. Balfour, Rockefeller Foundation Regional Director for the Far East, based in New Delhi, who was going to Chungking. They asked him to consult the PUMC Trustees in West China—Dr. Wong Wen-hao, Dr. Li Ting-an, and Dr. Y. T. Tsur—and advise the CMB as to what it might best do. When Dr. Balfour reached Chungking he found that these trustees had begun thinking about this question as soon as they knew the PUMC had been closed, and as early as February 28 had sent some specific suggestions to the CMB in a letter which did not reach New York until May 29. Even when on the same side of the line, wartime communications were often slow and unreliable.

Out of these various consultations, numerous lengthy letters and radiograms, and verbal reports to the CMB by Dr. Balfour whenever he returned to New York, the China Medical Board developed a wartime policy that the income of the Board should be "freely used" to help check the deterioration reported to be taking place in medical education in West China and "to strengthen the morale of medical teaching staffs and members of the student bodies" with "major emphasis... upon the clinical instruction of undergraduate students, postgraduate students, and nurses in the hospitals... but that attention be given also to the strengthening of premedical and preclinical education." It was also agreed that the size of the grants should be in keeping with the general scale of expenditures of the institutions aided, that funds should be appropriated as soon as possible, and held in New York subject to draft as needed. Since the PUMC Trustees had no legal power to act as a board except on PUMC matters, the CMB appointed a new "Wartime Advisory Committee" consisting of Dr. Wong Wen-hao, Dr. J. Heng Liu, Dr. Li Ting-an, and Dr. Y. T. Tsur (all PUMC trustees); Dr. C. K. Chu (a PUMC graduate), Assistant Director of the National Institute of Health; and Dr. Gordon King of the University of Hong Kong, then in West China. They also asked Dr. Balfour to represent the CMB in the Far East unless the program should grow to the point of interfering with his responsibilities to The Rockefeller Foundation.

During the course of the next three years appropriations totaling just over US$1,000,000 were approved, including some $445,000 for departmental aid in varying amounts to eight National Medical Colleges and two mission-supported institutions; about $200,000 for the re-establishment and operation in Chengtu of the PUMC School of Nursing, many of whose faculty and student body had made their way out of Peking; another $16,000 for emergency aid to medical and nursing staff and students of the PUMC in the southwest; $53,000 to the Commission on Medical Education of the Ministry of Education to support its endeavors to maintain standards; $47,000 for fellowship grants; $40,000 in discretionary funds for the field director to draw on for special needs of individuals; and approximately $100,000 to cover the cost of administering the program.

It soon became clear that the problems involved in administering this program called for full-time attention, something which Dr. Balfour's broad Rockefeller Foundation responsibilities did not permit. Accordingly, as of February 1, 1943, Dr. Claude E. Forkner was appointed Director of the CMB. Dr. Forkner had been Associate Professor of Medicine in the PUMC for five years in the mid-1930's, and he found many old friends and colleagues when he arrived in "Free China" in April 1943. He traveled extensively throughout the southwest, informed himself in depth about the various institutions and individuals asking for grants, and submitted well-documented recommendations which the CMB readily approved. As was inevitable under wartime conditions, challenging opportunities were all too often matched by problems and difficulties which militated against successful performance, a situation which Dr. Forkner found both distressing and frustrating. Like Mr. Greene and Dr. Houghton before him, he chafed under the tendency of the Board as supplier of funds to concern itself directly in matters of policy and program on which it might not always be as fully informed as the man in the field. His manifest frustrations notwithstanding, the two years he served as Director resulted in significant accomplishments for the CMB in helping to meet the immediate needs of medical education in "Free China" by conserving medical institutions and personnel disrupted by the war, and in facilitating the early resumption of the nationwide system of medical education and health services when the war was over. Unhappily, strong personality conflicts developed between Dr. Forkner and members of the China Medical Board which resulted in the termination of his active association with he Board in May 1945.

As of June 1, 1945, Dr. Balfour, with the consent of The Rockefeller Foundation, once again took over supervision of the CMB's wartime program, a responsibility which he carried until the end of the war called for liquidation of that program and a fresh look at future courses of action for the Board.

Chapter VII

LOOKING AHEAD

1943-1946

Outstanding Obligations

When the repatriation ship S. S. GRIPSHOLM arrived in New York on December 1, 1943, ten members of the faculty and staff of the College were among its fifteen hundred passengers.[*] The CMB was already busy with its wartime program, but the first order of business at that moment was to welcome and assist the returning internees. Cash advances and transportation home were immediately made available. The long-term obligations of the College would be studied as soon as the trustees available for discussion could be brought together in New York.

There were now seven trustees in the United States. Three had just returned on the GRIPSHOLM: Mr. E. H. Ballou, Chairman of the Executive Committee, Dr. A. M. Dunlap, and Dr. S. D. Wilson. Four had been here for some time: Mr. Arthur Bassett, Dr. Hu Shih, Dr. J. Heng Liu, and Dr. Sao-ke Alfred Sze. With three in southwest China—Dr. Li Ting-an, Dr. Y. T. Tsur, and Dr. Wong Wen-hao—ten of the eighteen duly elected members of the Board could now communicate directly with each other. The remaining eight in occupied China were, of course, inaccessible.

On December 16, 1943, just two weeks after the arrival of the GRIP-

---

[*] Dr. H. H. Anderson, Dr. J. L. Boots, Miss M. E. Ferguson, Miss E. H. Hirst, Dr. H. H. Loucks, Miss M. McMillan, Mrs. M. I. Pratt, Miss E. E. Robinson, Dr. F. E. Whitacre, Miss F. Whiteside, and Miss M. Wyne.

SHOLM, six of the seven trustees in the United States and the Secretary of the Board, met in a conference room of The Rockefeller Foundation. With them were Mr. Lobenstine and Miss Pearce, Chairman and Secretary of the CMB, and Dr. Loucks, named by the Shanghai Trustees in April 1942 to serve as *pro tem* Acting Director. Dr. Loucks and the Secretary of the Trustees, Miss Ferguson, were among the PUMC ten who had just been repatriated. Legally this meeting was "informal" since a quorum was not present, but no one was much disturbed since minutes would be recorded and any actions taken would be referred by mail to the other four accessible Trustees for comment and vote.

Dr. Loucks and Miss Ferguson reported briefly on the state of the Chinese members of the staff and of the property following the closure of the institution by the Japanese military, and told what they knew of the situation of Dr. Houghton and Mr. Bowen as of September 1943. The Trustees at the request of the CMB then turned their attention to the matter of the termination of appointments and liquidation of contracts. Fortunately minutes of the last meeting of the PUMC Executive Committee held in Peking on November 12, 1941, although fifteen months on the way to New York, were available for reference as the discussion proceeded. That was the meeting shortly before Pearl Harbor when the whole question of the contractual obligations of the College under existing circumstances and potential eventualities were extensively discussed, and a statement had been adopted outlining the general principles to be applied to the various categories of staff in the event of the closing of the institution.

It was now important to spell out the application of those principles as affecting the returnees and the liquidation of contracts of the increasing number of Chinese staff reaching southwest China. It was agreed that the general principles approved by the Executive Committee on November 12, 1941, should be reaffirmed as the basis for the termination of appointments and liquidation of contracts, with the understanding that in the case of Chinese members of the staff the term "salary" was to be construed as including subsistence allowances at the rate in effect on January 31, 1942, liquidated in U.S. currency at the rate of US$ 13.7 cents per FRB dollar (the currency of the Japanese-sponsored government in North China).

Thus was set in motion the long and sometimes complicated process of payments to more than 1, 200 persons. When the books were closed on

190

this undertaking on June 30, 1949, a total of US$230,229.80, provided for the purpose by the CMB, had been disbursed. Truly an outstanding instance of carrying out a moral obligation which legally might have been considered voided by the war.

Reconstituting the Board of Trustees

At the time this gathering of Trustees took place, Mr. Debevoise, Counsel to the China Medical Board, Inc., was concerned at the taking of actions which he described as "purely informal and of no legal effect or protection until ratified by a duly constituted quorum at a meeting duly called." There was, however, little prospect of getting the three trustees from southwest China to New York for a meeting with the seven presently in the United States, to secure a quorum. At the same time, there were many problems of personnel, policy and finance in the re-establishment of the School of Nursing in Chengtu, which needed definitive Trustee handling. Decisions affecting termination of contracts needed to be legally binding. Was there any way by which the Board of Trustees could be restored as a legal functioning body?

Mr. Debevoise was sympathetic with the problem, but thought the Trustees should have independent counsel, since the China Medical Board and The Rockefeller Foundation might have to ask him, as their legal adviser, to rule on the validity of requests made to them by the PUMC Trustees. He commended Mr. Sinclair Hamilton of the New York firm of Milbank, Tweed, Hope and Hadley. This was a happy choice for all concerned. Mr. Hamilton was intrigued by the somewhat unusual problems involved and with his assistants gave much thought to their solution.

The outcome was a petition to the Regents of the University of the State of New York from whom the College held its absolute charter, signed by the ten available Trustees, asking "removal for incapacity to act" of their eight fellow-trustees in Occupied China, and the appointment of three new Trustees to bring the Board to the minimum of the thirteen required. The Regents went through the statutory formality of mailing letters to each of the eight whose removal was being sought, informing them of the proposed action, and on September 15, 1944, "no objection having been made thereto or cause shown to the contrary" the Regents officially removed "because of their incapacity to serve as such Trustees" the group of eight in Occupied China: Keats S. Chu, S. J. Chuan, A. W.

Grabau, Sohtsu G. King, Lin Hsin-kwei, Bernard E. Read, T. A. Sun, and W. W. Yen. At the same time, they appointed Messrs. Li Ming, Charles R. Bennett, and C. C. Ch'en to serve until the Annual Meeting of the corporation in March 1947. The Trustees were once more a legal board.

No time was lost in calling the reconstituted Board together. On October 13, 1944, all nine of the Trustees resident in the United States met in the Board Room of The Rockefeller Foundation—two more than necessary for a quorum. One of their first actions was to record their high regard for those former colleagues who had been removed from office as a means of carrying on the work of the Trustees, and to express the hope that at some future date their membership on the Board might be renewed. Officers to serve until the Annual Meeting of 1945 were elected: Dr. Sze, Chairman; Dr. Dunlap, Vice Chairman; Miss Ferguson, Secretary; and a five-member Executive Committee composed of the four Trustees in southwest China, plus Dr. J. Heng Liu who, though based in Washington, might sometimes be in Chungking. Previous actions taken "informally" were ratified and thus made legal. The appointment of Miss Vera Nieh as Dean of the School of Nursing was confirmed. The appointment in Chengtu of a Committee on the School of Nursing was authorized. Problems of the School of Nursing budget, especially in terms of fluctuating exchange rates, were discussed. A committee of three Trustees was appointed to draft a statement in consultation with the officers of the CMB and The Rockefeller Foundation on postwar policy, for later consideration by the Board. In addition to the Executive Committee in Chungking, a Standing Committee of four of the Trustees resident in the United States was appointed to "transact such business of the Board as may arise... between meetings of the Board." The meeting ended with a graceful expression of appreciation to the CMB for all it had done for the College "during the period when the Trustees were unable to carry their own responsibilities." There was no question that the PUMC Board of Trustees was back on the job.

Although four of the five members of the Executive Committee were in Free China, it was no simple matter for them to meet. One was in Kweiyang, two in Chengtu, and one in Chungking. Travel was largely at the mercy of the military and a matter of priorities. A meeting was finally scheduled for March 1, 1945, in Chungking, but on that day only two were there—Dr. Wong Wen-hao and Dr. C. C. Ch'en. Once again it was necessary to disregard the fine points of the law, and in the interest of avoiding further delay in a number of matters of some urgency, Dr. Wong, outgoing Chairman of the Executive Committee, and Dr. Ch'en dealt item by item with the School of Nursing budget, the settlement of contracts of former PUMC staff in Free China, and other matters essential to the PUMC, keeping careful minutes and reporting all their actions by cable to the Trustees in the United States. When the Adjourned Annual Meeting convened in New York on March 24, 1945, with a quorum of seven Trustees present, they at once ratified and approved the actions taken by Dr. Wong and Dr. Ch'en. Once again unavoidable irregularities had been regularized.

At this meeting, the Trustees adopted the statement on the future of the College drawn up in consultation with the China Medical Board and The Rockefeller Foundation by the ad hoc committee appointed on October 13, 1944. The introductory paragraph expressed unqualified confidence in the reopening of the PUMC after the war. "The foreseeable future presents no less an opportunity for usefulness than did the years preceding Pearl Harbor." They recognized the fact that certain factors might temporarily or permanently affect the future of the College: the condition of the physical plant when the war was over; how best to fit into the Chinese Government's own national program of developing medical education, public health and medical research; the size of annual subsidy the CMB was prepared to give for the support of the College; and what new sources of income in China or abroad might be developed. While these and other factors prevented drawing up as yet an exact pattern for the College, the statement ended with a reaffirmation by the Trustees of their "purpose and determination to insure its reopening (together with the School of Nursing and the Hospital), the preservation of its professional work and academic standards at the same high level;" and a pledge "to seek continuously to discover fresh ways of promoting the aims for which the college was originally founded." This statement, widely publicized in China and in the United States, greatly encouraged the many who were interested in the PUMC's early postwar re-establishment. A group of medical missionaries meeting to discuss the future of their own programs, sent a heartwarming message to the Trustees recording their "very genuine appreciation of the contribution of the PUMC to medical education in China and to the work of many of our hospitals in giving postgraduate training;" and expressing their "earnest hope that this service can be re-opened and extended."

Planning for the Future

The determining role of CMB financial support in whatever plans might be made had been clearly recognized by the Trustees in their statement on the future of the College. Happily, the CMB was equally concerned about that future and believed that even though the war was not yet over, it was not too soon to begin a serious study of the factors involved. On May 31, 1945, at the CMB Adjourned Annual Meeting, an invitation was extended to the Trustees of The Rockefeller Foundation and those of the PUMC to appoint representatives to serve with CMB representatives on a "joint planning committee to consider what future steps may be taken for the advancement of medical education in China." The CMB members were Dr. Chester S. Keefer and Dr. H. B. Van Dyke, both of whom had once served on the PUMC faculty; Mr. Raymond B. Fosdick, Dr. Alan Gregg and Dr. Robert A. Lambert were the Foundation representatives; those appointed by the PUMC were Mr. E. H. Ballou, Dr. C. C. Ch'en, Dr. A. M. Dunlap and Dr. J. Heng Liu.

During the summer of 1945 there was much informal preliminary discussion in New York and in China. The presence of Dr. Houghton at the meeting of the Trustees on September 22, 1945, just eleven days after his return from four years as a prisoner of war, perhaps brought home more forcefully than all the newspaper headlines the fact that the war was really over, and that it was high time to think, talk, and act in specifics rather than generalities. Indeed at that very meeting the Trustees received a letter addressed to the President of The Rockefeller Foundation from Dr. T. V. Soong, President of the Executive Yuan of the National Government of the Republic of China, dated September 4, less than three weeks after V-J Day. This letter expressed the hope that the work of the PUMC would be resumed "at the earliest possible date" and that this would include not only the Hospital, but also the "immediate" reopening of the Medical College and School of Nursing so that "the important task of training Chinese men and women in the fields of clinical medicine, public health, medical education and research may be resumed." He pledged the cooperation of the Chinese Government "in every possible way to facilitate the resumption of this important work." This gratifying evidence of official interest together with Dr. Houghton's report of the widespread desire in Peking for early resumption of at least minimal clinical service, brought lengthy discussion. All agreed on the desirability of resuming as soon as possible some form of medical service even on a limited scale, a step which they believed would not prejudice any long-term recommendations from the Joint Planning Committee which had not yet met.

Certain preliminary steps were necessary whatever decisions might eventually be made. Mr. Bowen had already received the plant from the Japanese, in accordance with the authority delegated to him by Dr. Houghton before leaving, and needed a skeleton staff to maintain the powerhouse and other essential services. The Trustees accordingly gave Mr. Bowen specific authority to employ on a temporary basis such non-professional staff as might be required for this purpose. In addition he was authorized to start checking the inventory as far as that was possible, and to employ a temporary skeleton staff for the Library.

Dr. Houghton's report on the filthy condition of the buildings as he had seen them, led the Trustees to ask Miss Elizabeth Hirst, for many years in charge of the housekeeping services of the Hospital, to return to Peking as soon as she could conveniently do so, to work with Mr. Bowen in organizing the understaff for the extensive cleaning which the plant obviously required.

Since early personal contact with the Trustees in China, the Ministry of Education, and the National Health Administration, was highly desirable in any discussions and plans for the future of the College, the Trustees asked Miss Ferguson, Secretary of the Trustees and also Recorder of the College, to go to Peking as soon as possible provided such a visit would be in line with recommendations growing out of the forthcoming meeting of the Joint Planning Committee. It was also agreed that Dr. Loucks, then in West China on a State Department assignment, should be asked to visit Peking before his return to the United States so that his comments and advice would be available.

The Trustees had been dealing constructively with immediate problems but on a tentative basis only. When the Joint Planning Committee held its first formal session some two weeks later, October 9, the scope of its terms of reference were set out at the start by the Acting Chairman, Mr. Fosdick, around two broad questions:

1. What, exactly do we want to do in aid of modern medicine in China?

2. How can we implement our objective, once having determined what to do?

This made it possible to explore the situation from many angles and the discussion ranged widely and at length. It had not been expected that any conclusions would be arrived at in this first session, but the free and frank expression of opinions did result in a consensus that the CMB and The Rockefeller Foundation could probably do most for "the advancement of medicine in China" by concentrating their available resources on a single institution of high standard in Peking—in other words, by reestablishing the PUMC. The importance of further exploration of Chinese reactions and consultation in China with the Trustees and governmental authorities concerned precluded specific conclusions or recommendations at that time. Miss Ferguson's prospective trip should be useful from this viewpoint. The suggestion that it would be "highly desirable" that a survey of the situation be made on the ground, perhaps in the spring, by a group of qualified medical educators was left for later discussion. This ultimately led to the appointment of the Rockefeller Foundation Commission which was probably the most far-reaching result of the deliberations of the Planning Committee.

During the next few months while the various preliminary steps were being taken, consultations and discussions were for the most part informal as the individual members of the Planning Committee and others, who were interested in the developing situation, kept the various problems in their minds.

A letter dated November 26, 1945, from Mr. Fosdick to Mr. Rockefeller, Jr., who was always keenly interested in anything that concerned the PUMC, is of special interest in view of later developments:

One further point in relation to this whole question has to do with the additional funds which I hope the Trustees will be willing to vote to the CMB just as soon as the political and economic situation in China is straightened out. I think you and I have had in mind something like $6,000,000 to $8,000,000 to be added to the $12,000,000 which we gave the CMB in 1929. I retire as President two years from this coming June and I should like if possible to see this accomplished before I go. The work of the PUMC is among the bright jewels in our crown, and I think we have the strongest kind of obligation to continue our support of modern medicine in China.

Among the PUMC Trustees in China and in the United States, the chief subject of conversation was when and how to get the PUMC going again. A survey of the plant by a qualified engineer was seen as a matter of immediate urgency, the condition of the buildings and equipment having an important bearing on any plans for resuming activity. Equally urgent, they all agreed, was selection and appointment of a Director who could take part at the outset in the various consultations on the future of the institution, since Dr. Houghton would be retiring at the next Annual Meeting. The Chairman of the Trustees, Dr. Alfred Sze, began informally to gather suggestions as to possible nominees to succeed Dr. Houghton, and then appointed a nominating committee of three Trustees to present recommendations at a Special Meeting which he was planning to call for that purpose following the second meeting of the Planning Committee on January 16, 1946.

This meeting of the Planning Committee consisted for the most part of pooling information received from some of those who had gone to Peking since the first meeting in October. There was gratification at the word that the CMB had taken the first steps toward securing the engineering survey of the physical property of the PUMC (which all agreed was so essential in any long-term planning for reopening the institution). The question of sending a commission to China to study the PUMC and the implications of its re-establishment was again discussed, and it was agreed that the appropriate body to sponsor such a survey was The Rockefeller Foundation, especially since it was possible that the Foundation might consider increasing the endowment capital of the CMB to provide an income sufficient for the needs of the institution.

Dr. Houghton reported on the possibility of establishing an interim hospital unit at the PUMC under the auspices of the United Nations Relief and Rehabilitation Agency (UNRRA), which the CMB had asked him to investigate.

While this was being discussed, the meeting was interrupted by the arrival of a cable from Mr. Bowen reporting that, with the approval of Dr. Tsur, Chairman of the Executive Committee of the PUMC Trustees, and of Mr. T. A. Sun, a former member of the Board, he had made arrangements for housing at the College for a period of five months the Executive Headquarters of the tri-partite (American, Nationalist, Communist) Peace Commission headed by General George C. Marshall in Chungking. Although this might interfere with setting up the UNRRA hospital unit, it was agreed that the work of the Peace Commission was of such importance that it should have priority of consideration.

There was also some discussion of the perennial problems of RF-CMB-PUMC relationships with the hope that by the time the institution was again a going concern, past sources of misunderstanding and frictions might have been eliminated. In answer to an inquiry as to whether the Planning Committee was responsible for deciding such problems as the opening date of the College and the appointment of a PUMC Director, Mr. Fosdick replied that such matters were the responsibility of the specific boards, and that the Committee would consider only broad general policies and relations. No date was set for any future meetings, which would be called whenever pertinent information was received bearing on those matters for which this Committee was responsible.

In the course of the next few weeks there arose one of the unfortunate misunderstandings which unhappily cropped up from time to time in relationships between the home Boards and the PUMC Trustees. Dr. Sze believed that the RF and CMB had disclaimed all responsibility for the appointment of the Director which they considered the prerogative of the PUMC Trustees. Mr. Fosdick felt he had made clear to Dr. Sze that while this was undoubtedly the case, he thought it would be unwise for the Trustees to make an appointment while the Planning Committee and other inter-Board consultations were in progress and before basic conclusions had been reached. In any case, Dr. Sze had called for nominations from his fellow-trustees, and had set up a Special Meeting for February 23, for the specific purpose of appointing a Director.

When The Rockefeller Foundation and China Medical Board representatives on the Planning Committee learned that the PUMC Trustees were moving toward the early appointment of the Director, there was considerable surprise and perturbation. So strong was the feeling against an appointment being made at this time, that Mr. Fosdick assumed the distasteful task of writing to Dr. Sze suggesting the desirability of postponing the contemplated action. Dr. Sze replied at once in restrained language, which did not hide the shock and indeed resentment felt at this intervention, but stating that "in view... of the opposition reported by you and your own strongly expressed preference for delaying the appointment, I shall recommend to the Trustees at the meeting on the 23rd that action on the proposal to appoint a Director be postponed for later consideration." Once again the PUMC Trustees wondered how much real independence of judgment and initiative was theirs. When the Trustees did meet on

February 23, the only action taken on the appointment of a Director was the appointment of a committee consisting of Dr. Hu Shih, Mr. Ballou, and Dr. Wilson "to study the question of the Directorship and to make final recommendations to the Trustees."

One beneficial result from this otherwise unfortunate incident was the speeding up of action by The Rockefeller Foundation with regard to the proposed commission, which Mr. Fosdick realized was now imperative. On April 3, 1946, at the Annual Meeting of the Foundation, the Chairman was authorized to appoint a Commission to proceed to China and study on the ground the problem of the development of medicine and public health, reporting its findings and recommendations to the Board.

On March 27, 1946, the PUMC Trustees' Adjourned Annual Meeting was held in New York with the eight Trustees in the United States all present. Of these eight, five were hoping to return to China during the coming year; five were already there. The quorum would soon be on the other side of the Pacific, and in nominating officers and the Executive Committee this was kept in mind. Dr. Hu Shih was elected Chairman to succeed Dr. Sze; Mr. Ballou became Vice Chairman, and the Executive Committee consisted of the four Trustees already in China, plus Dr. J. Heng Liu who might occasionally be able to attend. The membership was held to the minimum of thirteen, but it was hoped that when regular meetings of the Board could be convened in China, the Trustees who had been removed from office in 1944 might once again be elected to membership. Having been informed by Mr. Fosdick that action on the proposed Commission would be taken on April 3, the Trustees deferred the election of a Director and decision on the date of reopening the Hospital and Medical School until after the Commission had made its report to The Rockefeller Foundation.

On April 17, the PUMC Trustees met in New York for the last time. This meeting like the Board's first postwar meeting on March 17, 1944, lacked a quorum and was therefore technically "informal." This was of no consequence, however, as the only purpose of the meeting being to hear directly from Miss Ferguson, who had just returned from China, no formal actions were called for.

When the Trustees next met on February 7, 1947, it was in Nanking, China, with four of the five members of the Executive Committee attending.

The Rockefeller Foundation Commission

Once the decision to send a commission had been made by the Foundation Trustees, no time was lost in its implementation. Dr. Gregg, as Director of the Division of Medical Sciences, was the obvious choice for Chairman. For the PUMC this was a particularly happy appointment for there was no one outside the institution who had so informed an appreciation of the significance of the enterprise and understanding of its problems. As early as 1933, after visiting the College for the first time he wrote: "It is probably of immense historical importance in the development of western medicine. In so huge a portion of the world's population, it is acting as a pace setter and a model, as a center of medical inspiration for Chinese physicians and foreigners in the Orient, and the optimum place for teacher training through the East." The other two members of the Commission, Dr. Sidney C. Burwell, Dean of the Harvard Medical School, and Dr. Loucks, who had been appointed to the CMB staff as of April 1, 1946, in the capacity of Representative, were each in his own way particularly well qualified to join Dr. Gregg in the desired survey.

A tactfully worded cable from Dr. Gregg to Dr. Y. T. Tsur, Chairman of the Trustees Executive Committee, reported the impending arrival of the Commission and asked him to inform the Minister of Education that they hoped for the benefit of his advice and consultation as they developed their report and recommendations in the field of medical education to the Foundation and the CMB. It was May 13 when the group arrived in Shanghai and July 22 when they left. During this time they visited Shanghai, Nanking, Peking, Kalgan, Chengtu and Chungking, with return stops in Nanking and Shanghai. Conferences were held with all available trustees, alumni and other individuals and groups, in government, education and business—Chinese and Western—observation at firsthand of damage to physical plants, losses in equipment, inadequacy of supplies, shortages in personnel, in schools and hospitals which were nevertheless operating as best they could—their time was filled to overflowing. Everywhere they went hopes rose that before too long there would once again be a functioning PUMC. But the members of the Commission did not forget that their terms of reference were "to study the situation in broad terms, not limited to the PUMC, nor to medical education exclusively, in order to present the needs of China that might properly be the concern of The Rockefeller Foundation and the China Medical Board and to aid

200

in the formulation of an effective program for the future."

During the summer, the members of the Commission worked on their report, individually and together, and in late September, Dr. Gregg gave Mr. Fosdick a copy of the report as it then stood—subject to further revision if this should seem desirable. The concluding summary of this draft of the report and recommendations started out with the statement that "China is now in a decisive stage of transformation... the possibilities and the opportunities in that country today are extraordinary... (The) needs... are so vast and so pressing that probably no private organization could be of effective help if it undertook a diversified and widely spread program. Selective emphasis on some one field is essential. The professional education of doctors especially for work in the field of public health and preventive medicine serves one of the most important needs of the Chinese people... and has the further advantage, already operative, of eager acceptance by the Chinese and a considerable part of its preliminary cost already paid in the form of buildings and experience at the PUMC. As a means of conveying humanitarian ideals, as well as the methods of scientific thought, medical education compares favorably with any other form of professional education."

The Commission went on to recommend "that The Rockefeller Foundation contribute to the support of medical education in China by further assistance to the China Medical Board, Inc.... that most of this support be directed toward re-establishing the PUMC and operating it as a medical school of high quality especially devoted to teacher training and the field of preventive medicine and public health; and that a definite proportion of this support be devoted to assisting other medical institutions in China."

To implement these general purposes, the Commission recommended: (1) appropriation by The Rockefeller Foundation to the CMB of additional endowment in the amount of $6,000,000, plus $3,000,000 in annual payments of $600,000 during the first five years of operation of the PUMC; (2) a reorganization of the CMB-PUMC relationships so that the PUMC Trustees should have full responsibility for the academic administration, educational policy and the management of funds received from the CMB and from other supporters; while the CMB would continue its present responsibilities associated with the guardianship of its endowment and the ownership of the land and buildings to be used by the PUMC. Finally the Commission recommended that "in the interests of mutual understanding the CMB contain always one Chinese member."

The report ended by expressing the "conviction that the time has come in the development of the PUMC for the transfer of responsibility and control, as above described. We believe this to be in the interest of sound administration and further adaptation to the Chinese milieu of that exceedingly complicated but precious service, a medical school of highest scientific and moral integrity."

Mr. Fosdick's first reaction was concern as to how these recommendations would be received by the Foundation Trustees who had not been thinking of such major financial provisions, particularly of transferring principal funds at that time. He consulted the financial officers of the Foundation, Mr. Walter Stewart, Jr., Chairman of the Board, and Mr. Rockefeller, Jr., no longer officially connected with any of the boards but with an abiding interest in the PUMC. They all seemed to feel that a terminal capital grant at that time would be unwise. The opponents of such action appeared to be very definitely in the majority. The members of the Commission had reason to feel that there was little chance of favorable action, but they continued to work on making their report as clear and cogent as possible in the hope that their own conviction of the importance of their proposals would in the end convince those who at first thought it too drastic.

In order to make sure that the report would receive the undivided attention of the Foundation Trustees, it was not placed on the docket of business to be taken up at the Annual Meeting scheduled for December 3-4 at Williamsburg, Virginia, but it was agreed after that meeting a Special Meeting of the Trustees would be called for the single purpose of dealing with the report.

In the meantime, Mr. Rockefeller, Jr., had been thinking back to the commitments he had made to the mission boards many years earlier when the institution was founded, and to what he had said to The Rockefeller Foundation Trustees on April 3, 1940, when he retired as Chairman of the Board. In his "Remarks" at that time he had spoken at some length about his pride in the record of the PUMC for which the Foundation had over the years made contributions in excess of $34,000,000. Referring to the fact that before the expiration of the five-year period covered by the most recent Foundation grant, the question of the relations of the Foundation to the future of the College would be coming up, he said: "It is the hope of your Chairman that if at that time world conditions justify, the Trustees will see fit to add to the present $12,000,000 endowment fund of the CMB, with the statement that that was its final gift and that the CMB and College must so plan as to operate on a self-supporting basis." He ended this part of his speech with an estimate that "any lesser sum than $5,000,000 would involve large sacrifices of existing values."

On returning from Williamsburg, Mr. Fosdick had called a meeting of the Executive Committee for January 16, asking Dr. Gregg to present the Commission's report, after which the question of a meeting of the full Board would be considered. With the call for the Executive Committee meeting went copies of the report which the members now saw in full for the first time. There Mr. Rockefeller found quoted what he had said on April 3, 1940, followed by the Commission's comment that "It has long been the expectation of the China Medical Board and the PUMC that such a terminal grant would be given. Not to make it would be a clear breach of faith both in China and in the United States." This was already much on his mind; and here his very words appeared again.

He was greatly impressed by the report as a whole, and so was Mr. Stewart, Chairman of the Board. They promptly conferred with Mr. Fosdick and together decided that the report should forthwith be placed before the whole Board, without preliminary review by the Executive Committee, and that all three members of the Commission should be invited to attend and present their case at a Special Meeting of the Board on January 16, 1947.

Most of the officers of the Foundation attended that meeting as well as Mr. Rockefeller, Jr., and the three members of the Commission. According to a contemporary account by Dr. Loucks, Mr. Fosdick opened the meeting by "reviewing very effectively the past history of the PUMC and CMB and their relationship to the Foundation, stated the reasons for sending out what he called the 'Fourth' Commission" and then gave the Commission the floor. Each one spoke. Dr. Gregg dispassionately presented the general basis of the recommendations, Dr. Loucks spoke about the actual accomplishments of the PUMC, and Dr. Burwell defended the cost. During the next hour and a half there was intensive discussion, with pertinent questions raised by various Trustees who were dubious about the proposals. According to Dr. Loucks, Mr. Rockefeller, Jr., was "the goal-keeper for the defense. Time after time he quietly, briefly, skillfully brought the discussion back to the original objective of developing an independent institution, the need to encourage and assign responsibility, the importance of removing uncertainty at this time, his own faith in the future. He would have given us 12 millions, and at one time it looked as though that was the amount we were going to receive. At other times, it looked as though a mere affirmation of future purpose would be the most we could expect. However, eventually the sum was fixed at 10 millions, as an outright grant and not as two separate grants, as suggested by the Commission."

Mr. Rockefeller had fulfilled his personal commitment.

The text of the resolution adopted at this meeting is so simple that no one would guess how much effort and heartache had preceded it:

RESOLVED that the sum of $10,000,000, be, and it hereby is, appropriated to the CHINA MEDICAL BOARD, INC., for its corporate purposes, payment of this appropriation to be made at such time in the discretion of the Executive Committee as the Committee shall consider proper.

Formal letters went that same day from Mr. Fosdick to the Chairman of the China Medical Board, Mr. Philo W. Parker; the Chairman of the PUMC Trustees, Dr. Hu Shih; to Dr. Alfred Sze, recent Chairman; Dr. Houghton, members of the Planning Committee, and others keenly interested in the PUMC. At the same time the good news was cabled directly to Dr. Hu Shih in Peking and to Dr. Y. T. Tsur in Nanking. The letters read:

The Rockefeller Foundation has today made a grant of $10,000,000 to the China Medical Board primarily for the support of the Peiping Union Medical College. This grant brings to $44,652,490 the sums which the Foundation has appropriated to the China Medical Board since 1915. Of this total sum, $9,804,999 was spent for the original land, buildings and equipment, $12,849,491 is the amount appropriated for the annual maintenance costs, while $22,000,000 represents the capital funds given the China Medical Board. This amount of approximately $45,000,000 is the largest grant ever made to a single project in the history of the Foundation.

In voting this appropriation today the Trustees of The Rockefeller Foundation wish to record the fact that it represents the terminal contribution of the Foundation to the China Medical Board and thus toward the work of the Peiping Union Medical College. Insofar as the Foundation is concerned, it completes the task undertaken in 1915, when the creation of a modern medical school in China was agreed upon. The development of new departments in the Peiping Union Medical College or further support of existing activities must be left to other friends of the institution. The Rockefeller Foundation can do no more.

In making an end to its contributions to the work of the Peiping Union Medical College, as they now do, and in withdrawing from the picture, the Trustees of the Foundation would again express their belief in this institution and in its high promise for the future. It has behind it a magnificent record of performance. Its graduates have introduced modern medicine into many parts of China. Its Trustees—and those of the China Medical Board—have served it with self-sacrificing devotion and loyalty. It has earned a unique name for itself in all the countries of the Far East. The Trustees of the Foundation are proud to have been associated in the founding of an institution whose contribution has been so significant and whose continuance means so much to the future; and they would take this occasion to rededicate it to the new generation of China in the firm belief that the light which it started in modern medicine will not be allowed to die out.

Through Dr. Sze in Washington, Dr. Hu cabled the appreciation of the Trustees at the Foundation action, adding that some time in February, after a full report had been received from New York, the Trustees would meet in Nanking to consider the appointment of a Director as well as the possible fall opening of the Medical School with first-year students only, together with a small hospital unit covering the four major services.

One final step remained—the windup meeting of the Planning Committee, which Mr. Fosdick had indicated to Dr. Sze should precede appointment of a Director by the PUMC Trustees. This meeting took place on January 28, 1947. Since the meetings in October and mid-January, Mr. Ballou, Dr. Dunlap and Dr. J. Heng Liu, three of the PUMC representatives on the committee, had returned to China leaving Dr. C. C. Ch'en, who was on a brief visit from China, the only one of the original four to represent the PUMC. Dr. Sze was also there on invitation of Mr. Fosdick. The meeting was informal, with a good deal of general but profitable discussion of what lay ahead. No attempt was made to take definite actions or to pass formal resolutions of any kind, since every question needing consideration was now, strictly speaking, within the jurisdiction of either the CMB or the PUMC. A cable went to Peking the day after this meeting reporting the dissolution of the Planning Committee.

The way was now cleared for the PUMC Trustees to assume and exercise their responsibilities.

Chapter VIII

BEGINNING AGAIN

1946-1949

Tʜᴇ ʟᴇᴛᴛᴇʀs from Mr. Fosdick and the China Medical Board officially confirming The Rockefeller Foundation grant to the CMB reached Peking in time to permit positive actions by the Trustees at the Annual Meeting on March 12, 1947, in Shanghai. At that meeting the Trustees took the first step toward the early re-establishment of the PUMC by appointing a Director, Dr. C. U. Lee.* They also recorded their hope that students might be admitted to the medical school in the coming autumn, with the Hospital reopening about the same time, while the School of Nursing and the Health Station would once again function as integral parts of the whole program.

The decision in early February by the tripartite Executive Headquarters to close out its activities in Peking, withdrawing all personnel, meant that whatever plans were developed for the PUMC could be based on the early availability of all the property for its normal purposes. The main build-

---

* At the same time, Dr. Alan Gregg was named Vice-Director, with the proviso that if a long-term appointment were not feasible, the Trustees would appreciate having him at the College for even six months. Touched by this expression of confidence, Dr. Gregg nevertheless felt he could not leave his responsibilities at The Rockefeller Foundation. The appointment was then offered to Dr. A. Baird Hastings, Professor of Biological Chemistry at Harvard, who had been a Visiting Professor at the PUMC in 1930-31, and was well known to Dr. Hu Shih, but he was unable to arrange for a leave. Although the Trustees still wished to have an American Vice-Director during the crucial years of re-establishment, no further appointments were offered because of the political situation.

ings were cleared in April and when Dr. Lee arrived on May 31 to take up his post, the last of Executive Headquarters personnel had just vacated Wenham Hall and the South Compound, leaving the PUMC free of all outside occupants.

Dr. Lee had been a member of the PUMC faculty for fourteen years, serving in the Department of Medicine until late 1937 when he crossed the lines into Southwest China to join in the anti-Japanese resistance. There he played a significant role under the difficult war conditions in maintaining medical education and services in "Free China." As Dean of the National Kweiyang Medical College, he won a reputation as a man with the qualities of integrity and leadership which the Trustees were seeking to set the tone of the reopened institution at a high level.

On his arrival in Peking, Dr. Lee turned at once to the arduous and time-consuming tasks that must be dealt with if the hope of re-opening the Medical School in the autumn of 1947 was to be fulfilled. Administrative machinery had to be set up, initial skeleton staff assembled, and budgets developed for both immediate and long-term (the CMB was asking for five-year forecasts) operation and rehabilitation. Pending major rehabilitation of power plant and shops, interim reconditioning must be undertaken as recommended in the preliminary engineering survey. Candidates for admission to the Medical School must be examined as soon as possible. Approaches to neighboring institutions for the cooperation that would cover the first-year teaching, brooked no delay. While assembling and sorting the conglomerate mass of equipment left by the Japanese, the staff should make every effort to secure a share of the supplies and equipment being distributed by CNRRA (the Chinese counterpart of UNRRA). The Library and clinical records, both of which were happily intact, must make room to receive the wartime accumulation of back journals held by the CMB in New York. Altogether it was a formidable job into which Dr. Lee threw himself heart and soul, developing a remarkable esprit de corps among his associates, everyone working tirelessly toward the realization of their common goal—the reopening of the PUMC.

Entrance examinations were given in Peking and Shanghai the first week in September to thirty-four candidates for admission to the Medical School coming from six different institutions, the furthest away being Fukien Christian University. Nineteen of these were accepted; and two who had been first year students in 1941 were readmitted. In October, just before the opening of the first trimester, one non-Chinese from Vancouver presented himself in Peking for examination, bringing to twenty-two the total number of students registered for the first year. Twelve of these already had B.S. degrees—there was to be no lowering of academic standards.

Formal instruction began on October 27 thanks to five exchange professors loaned by Tung Nan Medical College, Shanghai; Pei Ta Medical College; and Tsing Hua University. The course in gross anatomy started out with two cadavers "borrowed" from Pei Ta, soon increased to eight. Sets of histology slides had been salvaged from the piles of mixed and unidentified slides found here and there in the buildings. The students showed themselves as ready to adjust cheerfully to the makeshift conditions as were their instructors.

With the approval of the Trustees, the Dean of the School of Nursing, Miss Vera Nieh, had left Chengtu with a group of fifty students and staff on April 24 bound for Peking—a twelve-hundred mile trek on foot, by carts, bug-infested buses and trucks. It was mid-June when they reached Peking, to begin work on plans for reopening in the autumn. On October 1, sixteen students enrolled in the first year class. Since limitations of budget, equipment and supplies had made it impossible thus far to reopen any part of the Hospital, second and third year students had to look elsewhere for their clinical experience. The cooperation of the Central Hospital (Chung Ho), Hopkins Memorial Hospital of the Methodist Mission, and the Children's Hospital made it possible for the students to complete satisfactorily all the requirements for graduation and registration. Public health field work was fully covered at the First Health Station which had continued its service program throughout the war years, and was in addition, with the approval of the Trustees, extending its graduate teaching to classes of Health Officers and Tuberculosis Officers from the National Institute of Health in Nanking.

During the winter months the buildings around "C" Court were closed so as to conserve the limited and costly supply of available coal. Temporary quarters on the ground floor of "K" Building housed the administrative offices, but coal conservation was in effect there too, the boilers being fired only enough to keep the pipes from freezing. Those who worked in those offices during the winter of 1947-48 still remember their chill, with the indoor temperatures held in the low forties. The warmth of the Peking winter sunshine was never more appreciated than in those months.

When word of Dr. C. U. Lee's appointment as Director reached the China Medical Board, a cordial invitation was extended to him to visit the United States as guest of the Board, whenever it might be feasible for him to leave the PUMC for a few months. This greatly pleased the Trustees, as well as Dr. Lee who fully understood the importance of personal acquaintance with the officers and members of the CMB. By mid-December the academic year was well under way and the general rehabilitation progressing satisfactorily so that Dr. Lee felt he could be away from the College for a short time. He arrived in New York on December 28, spending the next two months in productive discussions, formal and informal, with new friends and former colleagues. He found such genuine interest and readiness to undertake the necessary support of the College that he returned to Peking greatly encouraged and, as he wrote Mr. Parker, Chairman of the CMB, with his "faith in the future strengthened immeasurably." The visit was equally encouraging to the CMB, many of whose members met Dr. Lee for the first time and found themselves in full agreement with the PUMC Trustees that the College was in good hands.

While Dr. Lee was away, the first welcome cash grants from the U.S. China Relief Mission were received at the College, as well as allocations of hospital equipment and supplies from CNRRA. These added to the fact that a careful financial review by Dr. Lee and his administrative colleagues showed operating costs substantially lower than anticipated, made it possible to open the first Hospital unit on May 1, 1948.

On that day there was a reception for the general public of Peking, who flocked in large numbers to visit the newly rehabilitated wards and laboratories. Many graduates of the Medical School and School of Nursing living in Peking joined the crowds. The beginnings were small: two wards of "P" Building (once the Isolation Pavilion) with twenty-five beds for general medical and surgical services only; the small operating room in the basement of that unit; outpatient service limited to fifteen patients a day in each of these two services. Small though it was, it was a welcome harbinger of more to come.

A special meeting of the Board of Trustees had been called for May 2 to celebrate this significant step forward in the restoration of the whole institution. A particularly happy circumstance was the presence at the opening reception and at the Trustees' meeting of Mr. Wm. Rogers

Herod, a member of the China Medical Board, who wrote back to New York enthusiastic impressions of the "capability and efficiency" of the staff who showed "evidence of being able to work as a team." Although he viewed military developments realistically and not without pessimism, he commented "I think it was wise to have gone ahead with the opening of the PUMC" and expressed the fervent hope that it might not be forced to close again.

The task of rehabilitating, re-equipping and restaffing the institution moved steadily ahead during the summer of 1948. The men medical students pitched in to prepare their dormitory, Wenham Hall, to receive the new class that would register on September 6. The women medical students moved from temporary quarters into the regular women's dormitory.

When the first trimester opened, each first year department was headed by a professor under regular full-time PUMC appointment. The dissecting laboratory in the Anatomy Building was back in use, with an adequate supply of cadavers. There were no more "borrowed" cadavers nor instructors "on loan." The regular student laboratories in "B" and "C" Buildings were also ready for the incoming first year class.

This was the encouraging situation which gladdened the hearts of medical and nursing graduates who gathered at the College on October 10, 1948, for their first Homecoming Day, an occasion initiated by Dr. Lee. But the Trustees and administrative officers were already keenly aware of increasing elements of uncertainty and apprehension in possible future developments, political and military.

The economic situation was giving the officers serious concern. The cost of living had risen sharply following the new economic regulations[*] announced by the Nationalist Government on August 19, which froze all salaries as of that date. By early October, living costs were eight times that level, and the Trustees Executive Committee approved a subsidy of 50% euphemistically called "winter relief," in lieu of salary increases. A further 50% was granted before the end of October, plus an additional

---

[*] These established a new currency, GOLD YUAN (GY), with a fixed exchange rate of GY4 to US$1 and called for prompt conversion at that rate of all foreign currency holdings with severe penalties against future possession of foreign currency. Many members of the PUMC staff promptly turned in the small nest-eggs of US banknotes which were their only savings against an uncertain future. When in less than three months the collapsing economy forced oficial revision of the exchange rate to 20 to 1, thus reducing the value of the Gold Yuan to 20% of its original value, there was widespread dismay followed by lack of confidence in the government's economic policies.

flat allowance of Gold Yuan 13 for those in the lowest wage grades. Even those subsidies were inadequate, but with exchange held at the official rate of GY4 to US1, the Trustees did not then feel justified in allowing more than that. In October the arrival of government flour rations for the previous six-month period provided each member of the staff with three bags of flour, which saved many from acute distress.

In November the Trustees raised the cash subsidy by another 50% plus a bag of flour bought on the open market by the Trustees. These actions would exhaust all then known savings by the end of December and put total salary requirements by January 1 to a monthly total almost twice the existing budget provision at the fixed 4 to 1 rate. Nevertheless the Trustees believed the action necessary to maintain the morale of staff and employees. Just after these actions, as the officers continued their never-ending review of the budget in search of further retrenchments, the government announced revision of the official exchange rate to 20 to 1. This greatly eased the immediate stringency and led to the hope that there could be a return to the "salary formula" based on the index of the cost of living. Even so there were other difficulties—there was a currency famine in Peking, and in addition the local branch of the Central Bank had not yet received official authorization to transact exchange at the new rate, an authorization that was maddeningly slow in coming.

There was at the same time mounting awareness of military developments and looming political changes. The 8th Route Army, the military arm in North China of the Chinese Communists, was drawing steadily closer to Peking. Military action between them and the Kuomintang troops of General Fu Tso-yi could easily occur.

The city was full of rumors; so too was the PUMC, but the morale of the staff and students was admirable. A few nursing students and members of the nursing staff were called home by families in the south. No medical students nor Chinese faculty left. The seven non-Chinese members of the staff all chose to stay on, the advice of their respective consular authorities notwithstanding, but the wives of two Americans did leave at that time.

On November 11, the Executive Committee, in response to questions raised as to the policy of the Trustees under existing circumstances, adopted the following statement for circulation to heads of departments and administrative units:

211

It is the desire and intention of the Trustees to carry on work as usual in Peiping, without any thought of moving away from this city. It is further their desire and intention to do whatever lies within their power to help the staff and students in any difficulties which may face them.

On December 4, the situation inside the city gates was sufficiently undisturbed for a cable to the CMB on routine matters to end with the familiar reassurance "All quiet here."

It was an illusory quiet. On December 13, the situation suddenly boiled up—and over. Firing was heard west of the city where Communist and Kuomintang troops clashed; the city gates were closed; the only transportation link with the outside world was a special plane, the *St. Paul*, operated ordinarily by the Lutherans to service their own missionaries, but now filled to overflowing by many, Chinese and Western alike, who managed to get on board, bound for some indefinite destination not yet under control of the Communist Army. Dr. Hu Shih and his wife succeeded in leaving the city that week, which left only two Trustees in the Peking area, Dr. Stanley D. Wilson at Yenching, already a no-man's land, and Dr. Chu Fu-t'ang in the city. Once again the PUMC officers were going to have to make decisions as the situation developed, hoping for eventual Trustee approval.

In New York the China Medical Board was watching developments anxiously, and on December 27 held a special meeting at which a formal statement of policy was adopted, which ended with reiteration of the "intention of this Board to continue to support the PUMC as long as, in the opinion of the Board, the PUMC can continue effectively to perform its mission in medical, hospital and educational work under the unrestricted direction and control of the present Director and staff, in whom the Board has every confidence, and whose loyalty to the institution and to high principles has been proven and tried."

In Peking, in spite of the generally deteriorating situation in North China, work was going along at the PUMC as usual: classes in session without interruption; the Hospital functioning to the full capacity of the 95 beds already in service and preparing to open another ward of 30 beds on January 3. The PUMC power plant and artesian wells made this possible at a time when the city as a whole was without its usual supply of water and light. On Christmas Eve, ten members of the Class of 1943 who had met all the requirements laid down by the Medical Faculty (having completed their work elsewhere but with no valid diplomas) were graduated at an all-College party in the Auditorium, ending with carols around the Christmas tree!

During most of January 1949, the Kuomintang troops of General Fu Tso-yi remained within the Peking walls, and those of the 8th Route Army stayed outside the city. No fighting of any importance developed and there was little damage from the occasional haphazard shelling. By the end of the month, a truce agreement had been arrived at and the Nationalist troops began to move out of Peking. Barbed wire came down, communications by air and rail reopened, and life in general returned to its normal pattern.

The Communist Army staged an impressive four-hour parade on February 3, in celebration of "Liberation Day," and the local populace responded with an enthusiastic welcome to the victorious soldiers who commandeered nothing, paid for what they bought, and were extraordinarily well-behaved.

Chapter IX

ADJUSTMENT TO
THE NEW POLITICAL REGIME

1949-1950

As CONDITIONS in the city and its surroundings settled down, the College kept moving ahead with its regular program. Rehabilitation of the hospital wards and clinics had proceeded so well that it was due to be completed by the end of February, except for some interior painting which was awaiting stocks of paint. The budget for 1949-50 was being prepared, and with resumption of rail communication with Tientsin, a quorum of the Executive Committee could meet together to consider it.

No official pronouncements had yet been made by the new government on educational policies in general, nor with respect to specific educational institutions like the PUMC, but unofficial contacts indicated according to Dr. Lee "an encouraging interest in the continuance of the College's function of training medical teachers and leaders, and a friendly concern that the buildings and equipment should be protected from harm." There was not yet any basis to forecast what future developments might bring.

Mails were none too certain although eventually most communications reached their destinations. Cable and radio service was reasonably regular, which made it possible to keep in touch with the CMB through weekly cables. One member of the staff commenting on the general situation wrote on February 17 "The messages that things were going on normally, that we were all undisturbed, that our financing was being handled in the usual fashion by drawing on our home resources, that the outlook was encouraging—all of these were not 'putting a good face' on the situation—they were plain statements of fact. If you could look in on us today I think you would be amazed at our complete normality. Offices all working as usual, committees meeting as frequently and lengthily as ever, outpatient department full of patients including orderly behaving members of the Liberation Army, hospital wards well filled, doctors, nurses and staff busy in their normal routines, students burning the midnight oil in preparation for the second trimester examinations which came last week at the scheduled time, and then going off to the Western Hills for a picnic to celebrate their brief spring recess."

There was as yet no official contact with the new authorities, no visitations or directives from their educational officers, although unofficial contacts were frequent and friendly with Chinese staff members. The lack of official contact seemed to be because there were too many other things of more immediate importance for the new authorities to attend to, and in the meantime they seemed content to let the College continue on its usual way. Everyone realized that many problems undoubtedly lay ahead, but at the outset it did not look as if they would be insoluble.

Dr. Lee showed himself an admirable Director through those difficult times, maintaining morale, and keeping everyone productively at work. In January, just as the political turnover was beginning, Dr. Lee initiated a series of twelve informal conferences with the Medical faculty. During that time of turmoil these served to keep them from losing sight of the main purpose of the College—medical education.

And so the weeks went by. On April 9, three members of the Executive Committee of the Trustees, constituting a quorum, met at the College for their first formal session since October 30, 1948—Dr. S. D. Wilson armed with a permit to come into the city from Yenching University, Mr. Keats S. Chu from Tientsin for the first time in many months, and Dr. Chu Fu-t'ang who lived in Peking. The two absent members, Dr. Hu Shih and Dr. J. Heng Liu, were both in the United States. Each had a long record of service under the National Government. During the course of the next few months both of them resigned from the Board of Trustees. Mr. T. A. Sun, a trustee but not a member of the Executive Committee, attended this meeting by invitation as did Dr. Loucks. Dr. Lee reported about the current difficulties in building up a permanent teaching faculty, mentioning among other things the absence of security when appointments had to be made on an annual basis, difficult traveling conditions for appointees with families coming from any distance, and the fact that the political situation nullified all efforts to secure visiting personnel from abroad. The result was that all departments were too thinly staffed and the teaching and clinical loads of the senior staff were too heavy. The hospital was expanding slowly but hospital receipts in relation to costs had shown a downward trend paralleling the progressive reduction of the paying ability of the community as a whole.

The formula designed to keep salaries and wages in line with continuing increases in the cost of living was not working as smoothly as in the previous year, but on the whole was keeping up with current living costs. Rehabilitation was approaching completion, and a tentative operating budget for the year 1949-50 within the limits of US$600,000 was reviewed and approved. How that year might be affected by external circumstances no one could foresee, but all were convinced of the importance of proceeding normally as far as possible.

During the spring the first movements came toward involving the PUMC in the city-wide unionization of teachers, students, clerical staff and understaff. There was no administrative opposition to these developments, but rather acceptance of the fact that this was a matter of personal decision for each one concerned. By summer there were four active organizations within the College—Students Union; Workers' Union; Clerical Union; and Professors' Union.

The China Medical Board was anxious to have Dr. Loucks return to New York as originally planned to take part in the budget discussions for the coming year, and to report on conditions at the College more fully than was possible by mail or cable. Although conditions in and around Peking were reasonably quiet, the Communist sweep southward was still in progress. It was the middle of May before Nanking and Shanghai were in Communist hands. This meant continued interruptions in travel, mails and cables. Dependable schedules were non-existent; stoppages were frequent and unpredictable, and periodically all communications were suddenly cut. In addition, exit and re-entry visas which were required for both Chinese and non-Chinese were not routine matters, but called for much time and patience, and even then might ultimately be refused. It had looked as if Dr. Loucks might not be able to get out of Tientsin before late May, but unexpectedly he was able to sail from there on April 24, reaching New York in time to report to a Special Meeting of the CMB on May 27. At that meeting in discussing the College budget, the members reaffirmed the policy adopted the previous December with regard to continued support of the PUMC, that the appropriation be paid on a quarterly rather than an annual basis.

Dr. Loucks was anxious to get back to Peking as soon as possible, but found it as difficult to accomplish as it had been to leave. It was September 5 before he finally arrived at the College to resume his full-time teaching and clinical activities in the Department of Surgery and to rejoin the small group working with Dr. Lee on the ever-growing administrative problems of the institution.

Mr. Bowen in the meantime had resigned as Treasurer, as of July 1, 1949, which he had been since May 1948 when the Trustees thought it was wise that the office of Controller which he had held hitherto, should be filled by a Chinese. He had planned to retire after seeing the rehabilitation program to completion, but the stresses and strains of the postwar period coming on top of four years under house arrest by the Japanese, and culminating in the difficulties with the labor unions during the spring and summer of 1949, had brought him to the conclusion that he could no longer be useful to the institution. The rehabilitation in which he had taken so keen an interest was far enough along so that it could be concluded by others. He was now ready to leave. The Executive Committee and Dr. Lee recognized the fact that the role of non-Chinese members of the staff would be increasingly difficult under the new regime, and agreed that he might go whenever he could get transportation. He left Peking on August 5.

Commenting on the labor situation which had triggered Mr. Bowen's resignation, Dr. Lee, in a letter to Dr. Loucks to New York dated July 8, gave an interesting analysis of general conditions in the new government administration. He pointed to the inevitable confusion and indecision even in the higher official quarters, where lack of experience was evident, "especially as applied to urban situations." He believed they were "deliberately tardy" in making decisions and adopting policies, hoping to gain time and experience before actually formulating rules and regulations. "In the meantime, institutional administration is necessarily very hit-and-miss." He spoke particularly about the confusion arising from failure to state clearly the difference from the union point of view between colleges and universities on the one hand and industrial plants on the other, although they recognized such a difference. Assuming that in the course of time such situations would be straightened out as new administrative techniques could be developed, at the moment it could fairly be said that "everything is in a state of flux, governmentally." The new authorities were not ready to give rulings on problems of administration of such institutions as the PUMC but, at the same time, former rules and regulations were no longer accepted as valid. He spoke of "the irksomeness of such a situation to us all, but especially to a man of Mr. Bowen's temperament. I have done what I could to hold him. I truly am sorry to lose anyone from our administrative group at this moment... Incidentally I think it is important to note that in my opinion his nationality has no bearing in this particular situation."

On Dr. Loucks' return to Peking, he found another hospital ward newly opened in August, and the Medical School preparing to receive 25 new first year students on September 12, the College's teaching program thus covering the first three years of the five year medical course. He also found the city in the midst of preparations for the formal establishment of the new government—the Peoples' Republic of China. Students and staff had instructions through their respective unions to get gray cotton uniforms following the accepted pattern, to be ready to participate in the city-wide parade and mass demonstration in front of the T'ien An Men on October 1—the new National Day with which the new regime replaced the "Double Tenth" marking the Sun Yat Sen Revolution.

Excitement mounted among the students. Detailed information on organization of the parade came from the Central Labor Union. All schools were closed so that everyone could take part. The PUMC contingent, which included students, workers, clerks and some professional staff (but not Dr. Lee), gathered in San T'iao Hutung between the Auditorium and "C" Court. While waiting for the signal to move, squad leaders taught them slogans to shout as they marched. It was evening before the last of the marchers saluted Mao Tse-tung and the other party leaders who stood on the balcony of the great red "Gate of Heavenly Peace" with its crown of imperial yellow tiles. This was the regime under which the future of the PUMC would have to be worked out.

In Dr. Loucks' first letter to New York after his return to Peking, he reported the whole institution "going ahead in a very normal fashion and the general morale of both staff and students high."

This letter was taken to New York by Miss Ferguson, who, with Miss Hirst, had left on October 13 on very short notice to embark on an un-scheduled freighter for Seattle on the "short leave" which Dr. Lee felt they both needed after the stress and strain of the past three years. Both women had been given re-entry permits and were due back in Peking February 1. Miss Ferguson also carried a letter from Dr. Lee to Mr. Parker which rounded out the picture of the situation as it had developed and presently stood.

Writing on October 12, 1949 Dr. Lee described the first months after the "liberation" of Peking as a period of marking time, waiting for policies to be announced so that the College's plans could be framed accordingly. "We often felt we were working in the dark." The intensive preparation for the People's Consultative Council (PCC) had extended beyond "strictly political circles" into all walks of life. "This was the time when labor problems began to loom up, when our workers' union was formed... to begin with the workers were more concerned with what they could get than with their particular contribution to the development of the institu-tion... but after... strenuous efforts... to find a reasonable meeting ground, there are signs of a dawning consciousness... that each person in the PUMC has a responsibility toward the institution. The period of the PCC meetings was one of carefully fostered and mounting enthusiasm, rising to the climax of the great mass meeting on October 1, when the establishment of the People's Government of the Republic of China was celebrated."

Dr. Lee went on to remark that the current program of the College and Hospital was proceeding normally without interference, but plans for the future were still awaiting formulation of policies by new ministries not yet established. There was considerable evidence, however, that "the con-tribution of the PUMC in concentrating on quality rather than quantity" was appreciated, and might be encouraged as an important element in forthcoming plans for "medical education and health services for the whole people."

Commenting on his own attendance at the PCC meetings as one of the medical representatives elected by the All-China Science Association, Dr. Lee said he had not been happy at his election, since in the past he had always avoided political activities. As it turned out, however, it had given him a useful opportunity to meet many people from other parts of China, including old friends, and had not interfered with his duties at the College. To his satisfaction he had not been put on the continuing committee of the PCC so his "unsought excursion into the political field" was over, but he believed that his participation in the PCC had strengthened the independent position of the College because of the opportunity it gave him to explain the institution's purposes.

In conclusion, Dr. Lee wrote "Changes of great magnitude have taken place in the past year, but I sincerely believe that there is still an important place for the College in the field of medical education and service in China in terms of the high purposes of the founders."

At the Adjourned Annual Meeting of the CMB in New York on November 14, 1949, these letters were at hand for consideration. Mr. Fosdick had been invited to attend in his capacity as a member of a special committee on Far Eastern affairs in the Department of State. According to the Minutes, the U.S. Government was in favor of continued support of such institutions as the PUMC, having every desire that American contacts with China be maintained as long as possible, particularly in the missionary and educational field. Once again the CMB made clear that the support of the College would be continued as long as the College was under the administration of Dr. Lee and conducted in accord with the policies and ideals for which it was originally created, and without undue interference from the Chinese authorities which would make it impossible to carry out such policies and principles.

The members of the Board, however, were not unmindful of the fact that restrictions might be placed on the PUMC at almost any time and that it would be impossible for it to continue functioning and for the Board to continue support. The Chairman suggested the advisability of beginning to think about possible substitute programs in such an eventuality. The Board responded favorably to Dr. Loucks' proposal that the CMB assume responsibility for the US$ salaries of the present foreign staff of the College as an emergency measure on a year-to-year basis— generously covering this over and above the $600,000 for the operating budget.

Before leaving Peking, Miss Ferguson had been asked by the Trustees to consult the CMB and its counsel on restoring the name of the institution to the Peking Union Medical College, the name of the city having

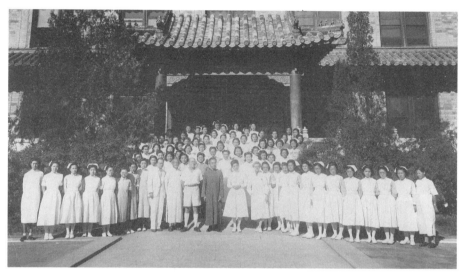

School of Nursing returns to Peking—September 6, 1946
(Miss Nieh and Dr. Hu Shih are in center of front row.)

The Reopening of the Hospital — May 1, 1948

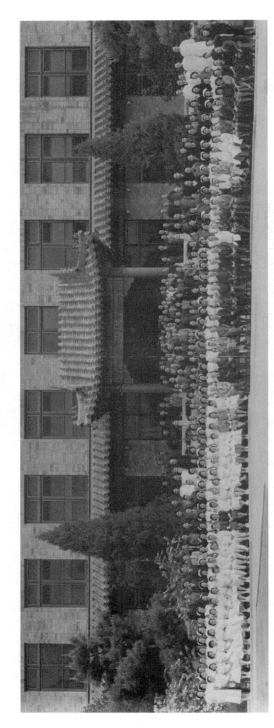

Center of front row — Trustees and administrative officers with Mr. Wm. Rogers Herod representing the CMB.

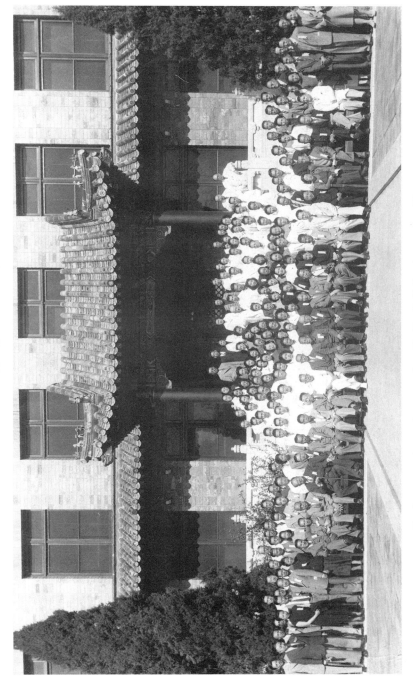

Homecoming Day — October 9, 1949

Graduates, undergraduates and staff — Dr. C. U. Lee in center of front row.

Minister of Education and Head of Department of Higher Education visit the College—October 6, 1950

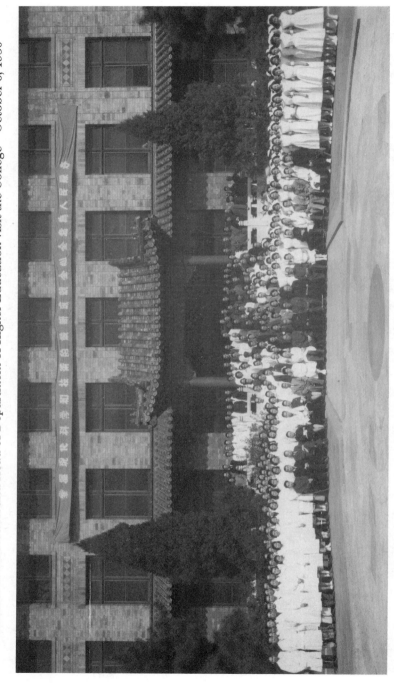

Overhead banner reads: Now in control of the newest achievements in science and technology to put to the service of the people wholeheartedly. (This is the last picture received from Peking.)

reverted under the new regime from *Peiping* to Peking. The CMB counsel saw no objection to instituting formal action by the Regents of the University of the State of New York, and in the interim using the new name on letterheads and bank accounts, a fact which was cabled at once to Dr. Lee. On December 11, 1949, the Executive Committee in Peking approved the immediate change, bringing the name of the College full circle back to that adopted when it was incorporated in 1915.

Three PUMC Trustees in the United States, all *persona non grata* to the Communists, had resigned in recent months; Dr. Stanley Wilson had returned to the United States, and current travel restrictions made it impossible for Trustees from the Shanghai area to attend meetings. This left the responsibility for the orderly conduct of the Board on the three who happened to live in Peking and Tientsin—Mr. Keats S. Chu, Dr. Chu Fu-t'ang, and Mr. T. A. Sun. Dr. Lee and others in the administration were meticulous in consulting them, presenting the budget as usual for consideration, submitting current financial reports on operation and rehabilitation, discussing with them the mounting difficulties in the new situation, and as far as possible keeping them in touch with developments and actions in New York. This was one more evidence—the uncertain situation on both sides of the Pacific notwithstanding—of the strong determination to carry on normally as long as possible.

As the time approached for Miss Ferguson and Miss Hirst to return to Peking, there arose within the CMB some concern as to the wisdom of their doing so, particularly on the part of Mr. Herod, one of the few CMB members with personal business experience in China, apart from Mr. Parker, the Chairman, who happened to be in Europe at that moment. Mr. Herod knew of the difficulties many business firms were having in getting permits for their "foreign" employees to leave China, especially in the Shanghai area where the heads of many companies were being held virtually as hostages against payment of large sums allegedly owed for unpaid taxes or other unusual charges. In the absence of Mr. Parker, Mr. Herod took the question up with Dr. Hinsey, Chairman of the Executive Committee, and together they assumed the responsibility of asking these two women not to return to Peking without securing release from the CMB. This action brought prompt objections from Dr. Lee and Dr. Loucks as well as pleas from the two directly affected who were anxious to get back to relieve the small group in Peking who were carrying their work in addition to their own. These protests notwithstanding, the CMB maintained its stand, which by summer was extended to questioning the wisdom of allowing *any* American staff, including Dr. Loucks, to remain at the College under existing conditions. Dr. Adolph, Professor of Biochemistry, had already planned a brief visit to the United States during the summer, which would leave Dr. Loucks the only American at the PUMC. Wishing to avoid the appearance of giving instructions to persons under appointment by the PUMC Trustees, the CMB asked its own appointee, Dr. Loucks, to come to New York "to report on conditions in Peking"; asked Miss Ferguson to defer departure for Peking pending Dr. Loucks' arrival; and Miss Hirst, who was already in Hong Kong, to return to the United States so that all three might participate in the coming discussions in New York.

Dr. Loucks was reluctant to leave Peking because it would further reduce the number of colleagues available to share Dr. Lee's heavy administrative load at a time when the special problems of dealing with the new officialdom were especially time-consuming and onerous. He concluded, however, that direct discussions with Mr. Parker and the members of the Board might clarify the situation sufficiently for the CMB to agree to lift the ban on the return of those Americans who wished to resume their posts. By good fortune he secured passage on the same ship on which Dr. Adolph was sailing the end of June, and was in New York a month later.

His first meeting with Mr. Parker and the other members of the CMB Executive Committee was on August 4. Dr. Loucks realized that the North Korean invasion of South Korea and other developments, including the appointment of General Douglas MacArthur as Commander of United Nations forces in Korea, which had occurred since he left Peking, meant that until the Korean situation was resolved (which most people assumed would be within a few months at most) the CMB was not likely to agree to the return of the PUMC Americans to that side of the Pacific. He found Mr. Parker and other members of the Board sufficiently sympathetic to the situation in Peking, however, to hope that by late autumn he and Miss Ferguson might be allowed to return to the College.

In the interim he devoted himself to frequent talks with individual members of the CMB, laying before them a picture of the postwar accomplishments of the College, describing the complexities of adjusting to changing external circumstances and pressures while maintaining with surprisingly little interruption the normal program of teaching and hospital service, and developing their appreciation of the reasons why he and his American colleagues were so anxious to return to help the institution and its Chinese staff through this time of trial. He also kept in close touch with Dr. Lee by letter and at Dr. Lee's request, concerned himself with various College matters—personnel, books, shipping problems, insurance of the buildings, the needs of the power plant.

For all four—Dr. Loucks, Dr. Adolph, Miss Hirst, Miss Ferguson— these months were basically a time of suspense, anxiously following the news, listening on the radio to sessions of the Security Council of the United Nations, spirits rising when the Korean War seemed to be moving toward an early and successful conclusion, and waiting for November 8, the scheduled date of the CMB meeting at which there began to seem a real possibility that the Board members would give them their release. TIME magazine, in its issue of October 16, commented: "Only a Chinese Communist or Russian army marching to the aid of the Korean comrades could possibly stave off a swift defeat for the Red aggressors. But, more and more, such intervention seemed unlikely." The last week of October saw the fall to U. N. forces of the North Korean capital, Pyongyang. Again quoting TIME in its issue of October 30: "Now that the war was ending" the problems ahead were those of reconstruction. So hopeful was the PUMC group in New York that they had quietly made reservations on a ship due to sail from San Francisco on November 27, so that if their return was cleared on November 8 they could be on their way promptly.

The first week in November brought a complete reversal of the situation in Korea, with massive attacks throughout northwest Korea and along the banks of the Yalu River spearheaded by large numbers of Chinese troops brought down from Manchuria. To the four who had been so confidently awaiting the CMB meeting, it was painfully clear that talk of return by any of them at this moment would be futile. It was now for the CMB to consider seriously the effect of these new developments on its relationship to the College, and to prepare for the possibility that external circumstances might at any time bring about an abrupt end to that relationship.

It was in this context that the members of the CMB met on November 8 to review the total situation facing them. There was no suggestion of panic, and no one seriously questioned a continuation of the CMB's expressed policy of support for the College. There was no change, however, in the Board's position on the return of the American staff members at that time, the four affected taking meager comfort from the assurance that the Executive Committee would give sympathetic consideration to the question whenever the skies seemed to be clearing again. Approval in principle of the purchase of the greatly needed new boilers for the power plant in Peking whenever this might be practicable, was tangible evidence of the strong hope of everyone that the CMB bonds with the College would hold fast.

The day after the meeting, the PUMC four cancelled the steamship reservations so optimistically made a few weeks before, and turned to thoughts of their own immediate futures. Grievously disappointed as each was, they realized that there was little foreseeable prospect of returning to Peking. The only consolation in not being there to help their Chinese colleagues as they faced increasing governmental pressures on policy and program, was that Dr. Lee's problems might be simplified by the fact that they were *not* there. "The complete absence of Americans from your midst" wrote Dr. Loucks to Dr. Lee "may be a blessing rather than otherwise."

This feeling led Dr. Adolph, Miss Ferguson and Miss Hirst, after consultation with Dr. Loucks and the CMB, to write to Dr. Lee each resigning from their posts in the College as of November 30, 1950. For Dr. Loucks this was not necessary since his appointment with the College was that of an unsalaried Visiting Professor of Surgery, his substantive appointment being under the China Medical Board as Representative.

Chapter X

THE LAST DAYS OF
THE OLD ERA

1950-1951

ONE fortunate circumstance just before Dr. Loucks left Peking was the appointment of Mr. Sun Pang-ts'ao as Recorder and Acting Chief of the Secretariat beginning July 1, 1950. It was a great satisfaction to everyone to know that Dr. Lee had the highly qualified Mr. Sun to relieve him of many administrative routines, to carry on a large part of the English language correspondence, and to keep minutes and other records up-to-date. As the months went by, Mr. Sun's informative and often witty weekly letters to Miss Pearce together with letters and cables from Dr. Lee, kept the absent staff members and the CMB remarkably close to the College and aware of continuing and expanding activity in spite of the abnormal and unpredictable atmosphere in which they were carrying on.

Thirty-three candidates for admission to the Medical College took the regular entrance examinations in the summer of 1950, of whom twenty-five were accepted. The College could still maintain its existing requirements for admission for the Ministry of Education had indicated that no change in the entrance requirements was as yet contemplated, although a proposal for shortening the medical course to five years, including premedical sciences, had already been made for all medical schools. The School of Nursing also accepted twenty-five applicants for the first year. The enrollment of fifty new students appeared to satisfy the recent suggestion of the Ministries of Health and Education that if possible the

PUMC admit a minimum of sixty new students. The applicants for admission came from eight colleges and universities, five of which were outside North China—Soochow University, Fukien University, St. John's University (Shanghai), Ginling College (Nanking), and Wuhan University (Wuchang)—all institutions from which the College had drawn students in the past. Training courses in the Hospital which had already produced six dietitians and five social workers, enrolled further trainees.

During the summer the routine program of exterior painting of the buildings was in progress. Coal was contracted for the whole year at about US$5.50 a ton. The plans for purchase and installation of the two big new boilers to replace the existing ones were worked out for Trustee consideration in time for CMB action on November 8. On July 20, the Executive Committee of the Trustees met at the College, dealing in the usual fashion with reports and recommendations of the Director. They were told that the College was definitely under the jurisdiction of the Ministry of Education (not the Ministry of Health as had been feared) and that it was necessary for the College to be registered with this Ministry. This was not the first time that the Trustees had to study regulations to see what changes in the existing structure were needed to comply. The outstanding problems were "a properly constituted Board of Trustees," Chinese control of finances, and transfer to Chinese control and ownership of the properties and other physical assets. According to Mr. Sun's minutes the Trustees "took the view that the difficulties indicated were not insurmountable." A Nominating Committee was appointed to fill the vacancies resulting from resignations and absence abroad of a significant number of Trustees during the past year. The CMB appropriation of US$600,000 for the operating budget for 1950-51 was acknowledged with appreciation, note was taken of the officially required contribution of 2% of the payroll to the College Labor Union, there was preliminary discussion of various proposals for the investment of the Retirement Savings Account—the Trustees were doing their part in carrying on "as usual."

Four national conferences were held that summer of 1950 at the PUMC—the China Medical Association, the Chinese Nurses Association, a conference on Public Health, and one on Science. Dr. Lee and members of the PUMC faculty played an important part at these meetings, as did PUMC graduates coming from other institutions.

On the evening of August 22, the graduation of twenty from the School of Nursing was celebrated by a buffet supper in "C" Court at which altogether 154 graduates of the PUMC were present, every class since 1924 (the first class) being represented, plus one graduate (1919) of the old Union Medical College.

One innovation during the summer was a weekly series of eleven Clinical Pathological Conferences for the medical workers of the city held by Dr. C. H. Hu, Professor of Pathology, at the request of the Ministry of Health. Mr. Sun wrote of "their unqualified success and popularity. The extraordinary enthusiasm of the audiences is difficult to account for, unless it be that Peking affords too few amusements... The Auditorium has been packed to overflowing with never less than 500 people attending, jamming the doorways and blocking up the windows. The Ministry of Health... has requested the publication in book form of all the proceedings. Even sound movies have been suggested." And to Dr. Hu's satisfaction there was developing as a result an increase in the number of autopsies secured.

When the first trimester opened two more clinics were in service— otolaryngology and ophthalmology—so the fourth year students would not miss work in these two specialties. Mr. Sun commented "the College is a veritable beehive of activity. It is pleasant to see so many young people about and to hear their gay laughter."

On September 23, the Executive Committee of the Trustees received the Controller's financial report for 1949-50 and the auditors' report for the same period, together with the reports for 1947-48 and 1948-49 which had been delayed by the inability of the Shanghai-based auditors to get to Peking. It was decided to hold a General Meeting of the Trustees in Shanghai later in November or early in December, if possible. In preparation for that meeting, Mr. Chu, Mr. Sun and Dr. Chu, acting as a Nominating Committee, began discussing possible candidates for vacancies in he Board Membership.

Much of Dr. Lee's time had to be spent on extra-mural activities, which he wrote had given him "wider contacts and new experiences... And I have the comforting feeling that perhaps at this stage the Chinese people require above all things strict social discipline, greater sacrifice and more hard work." Speaking of the difficulties in rebuilding the faculty and adding to the new equipment needed for development, he voiced the earnest hope "that the international situation will soon improve so as to allow our colleagues to return at an early date and the continuance of our high quality of training and service."

Homecoming Day was celebrated on October 7, with more than 100 graduates of the Medical College and the School of Nursing in attendance. as well as a large number of faculty members, past and present. There was special interest in the fact that on the day before, the Minister of Education and the Head of the Department of Higher Education had visited the College. After speech making in the Auditorium and a group photograph in "C" Court, there was a round of inspection. Mr. Sun reported that both speakers urged the PUMC with its high quality in teaching and service "to carry out the government's health and education programs and extend its usefulness for the benefit of the people." Mr. Sun wrote that there was no question that "the standard we set is appreciated."

Along with satisfactions such as these, there was no lack of problems. Labor relations and wage scales were matters of almost continuous concern. There were by then two unions in the College—the Labor Union and the Educational Workers Union, with the former dominant at least as far as numerical representation went. Members of the administrative staff might sit in on the Preparatory Committees and Working Committees which considered such things as salary adjustments, but whether simply as observers or in any more substantial capacity remained to be seen.

Eventually as a result of many meetings and much discussion, a relatively simple plan was worked out which was gratifying evidence of the continuing confidence in the administration by all concerned. In actual practice there was no significant change in the established procedure, except to provide that increases in salary would be decided upon by the Salary Adjustment Consultative Committee composed of members of the administration and representatives of the unions.

A more difficult and ticklish situation was a request from the Ministry of Health (Weishengpu) for temporary occupancy of a part of the hospital (250 beds) to be used for government employees needing hospital care. A similar request was being made of other hospitals in the city. The Ministry's own construction program had been delayed and beds were immediately needed for the many sick workers in public employ who were paid on a maintenance basis including sick benefits.

After consultation with the Ministry of Education and his colleagues in the faculty, Dr. Lee concluded that this request must be met. He hoped that good would come out of the arrangement—such as daily contact with Weishengpu personnel, and the high ranking officials who as patients would get a better understanding of the work of the College. The Weishengpu representatives were insistent that there should be no impairment of the PUMC standard of teaching and service. Dr. Lee hoped that he was not being unduly optimistic for he knew difficulties and possibly frictions were bound to arise, but he was in a situation where he could not refuse the request and he looked for understanding from the CMB.

As December wore on, letters and cables on both sides of the Pacific dealt as far as possible with matters of immediate concern, but underlying all these efforts to keep things going, there was increasing despondency over the course of events. On December 18, the U.S. Treasury Department officially froze all financial transactions with China, and all bank accounts having any connection with China. Dr. Loucks and the members of the CMB immediately began exploring possibilities for getting special licenses for remittances to the PUMC, but with little hope of success. A shipping embargo was placed on goods destined for Communist China. Mails and cables continued to get through without undue delays, but there was little from either end that was encouraging to report.

The end of December brought counter-freezing of American assets in China. On December 28, the CMB Executive Committee met to consider the situation as of that date. The atmosphere was very pessimistic as there seemed little possibility of securing the license needed for the College to draw funds from its account in the National City Bank, or for the Board to provide new funds for use by the College. Specific permission was required for the CMB to pay bills on behalf of the College, and such permission was hard to get. It would be even more difficult to get a permit for general support. Nevertheless, every effort was made, every possibility explored, in the face of the unwelcome fact that the time seemed fast approaching when the CMB would no longer be able to send any financial support. The Board fully appreciated the fact that when that time should come, the College would have no alternative but to turn to the government, a fact which in no way lessened the Board's confidence in the administration and staff of the College.

On January 2, 1951, Mr. Sun wrote the last of his weekly letters to be received in New York—letters which had played so important a part in maintaining close touch with developments in Peking. He was leaving that afternoon with Dr. Lee and Mr. James Ch'en, Controller, for Shanghai to attend the Trustees meeting which had been postponed so many times. They expected to get back to Peking on the 10th.

On January 17, Dr. Loucks cabled to Dr. Lee (cable #51001) in reply to an inquiry about the possibility of remittances to the College, saying: "No decisions reached but not without hope. Board meeting January twenty-four. Any possible prior reassurance worthwhile."

In a covering letter of that same date he wrote to Dr. Lee explaining that word had come through "that the first hurdle had been cleared as far as a permit to unfreeze a portion of the College funds in the National City Bank is concerned. The permit, if it finally is effective, will be for only one-half the amount requested in your original cable, but we know how much even this amount will mean... Much will depend on such assurance as we can give the CMB and other interested individuals as to the progress of events at the College..."

"... I now merely want to add the hope that, if we can secure final approval for the unfreezing order, the Board also may be willing to apply for license for the regular remittance of funds. I am most skeptical as to whether it will be possible to remit funds as large as those formerly sent, but we hope that at least sufficient funds to meet your regular payrolls, and perhaps the most necessary supplies can be provided. All of this, however, is certainly more nearly in the realm of wishful thinking rather than that of accomplished fact at the present moment."

On the morning of January 23, 1951, Dr. Lee's cabled reply came to the China Medical Board:

REFERRING YOUR 51001 COLLEGE NATIONALIZED JANUARY TWENTIETH

This was the last direct word from the College.

The long and productive years of CMB-PUMC cooperation had ended.

EPILOGUE

Wɪᴛʜ You, I deeply regret that the Peking Union Medical College should have passed out of the hands of the China Medical Board and been taken over by the Peking Government. However, I presume this was inevitable and that it was only a question of when the seizure would take place.... We must not feel that this necessarily means a curtailment of the College's usefulness, but rather only a change in its management attended very probably by certain limitations in its ideals and standards. But who are we to say that this may not be the Lord's way of achieving the intent of the founders, although it be a way so wholly different from what has been in our minds. Let us hope, pray and believe that all may be ultimately for the best.

JOHN D. ROCKEFELLER, JR.
writing to a friend
April 4, 1951

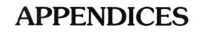

APPENDICES

TRUSTEES OF PEKING (PEIPING)
UNION MEDICAL COLLEGE
1916-1951

MEMBERS

Armitage, James Auriol	1918-1924	Li, T'ing-an	1936-1948
Ballou, Earle H.	1936-1948	Lin, Hsin-kwei	1933-1944
Barton, James L.	1918-1929	Little, L. K.	1947-1950
Bassett, Arthur H.	1940-1948	Liu, Jui-heng	1929-1949
Bennett, Charles R.	1929-1939,	Lobenstine, E. C.	1929-1936
	1944-1947	Monroe, Paul	1920-1925,
Brown, Arthur J.	1918-1929		1928-1931
Buttrick, Wallace	1918-1926	Mott, John R.	1918-1927
Chang, Po-ling	1929-1938	North, Frank Mason	1918-1929
Ch'en, Chih-ch'ien	1944-1950	Pearce, Richard M.	1928-1929
Chu, Fu-t'ang	1948-	Read, Bernard E.	1936-1944
Chu, Keats S.	1940-1944, 1951-	Reid, James Christie	1918-1926
Ch'uan, S. J.	1938-1944	Rockefeller, John D., Jr.	1918-1929
Cochrane, Thomas	1926-1929	Rose, Wickliffe	1918-1919
Dunlap, A. M.	1939-1951	Sellett, George	1948-1951
Fang, Shisan	1935-1941	Sun, T. A.	1941-1944, 1947-
Flexner, Simon	1918-1929	Sze, Sao-ke Alfred	1926-1948
Grabau, A. W.	1938-1944	Thomas, Charles F.	1948-1949
Greene, Roger S.	1922-1938	Ting, V. K.	1932-1937
Hawkins, Francis H.	1918-1929,	Tsur, Y. T.	1929-1950
	1931-1935	Vincent, George E.	1918-1929
Houghton, Henry S.	1935-1940	Weir, H. H.	1924-1929
Hu, Shih	1929-1949	Welch, William H.	1918-1929
Hubbard, G. E.	1929-1933	Wilson, Stanley D.	1941-1949
King, Sohtsu G.	1930-1944	Wong, Wen-hao	1929-1950
Kirk, Robert H.	1919-1921	Wu, C. C.	1929-1933
Li, Ming	1944-1951	Yen, W. W.	1930-1934,
			1940-1944

PRINCIPAL OFFICERS

CHAIRMEN

John R. Mott	1916-1920	Y.T.Tsur	1929-1939
Paul Monroe	1920-1926	Sohtsu G.King	1939-1944
Sao-ke Alfred Sze	1926-1929, 1944-1946	Hu Shih	1946-1949

SECRETARIES

Wallace Buttrick	1916-1918	Margery K. Eggleston	1927-1932
Edwin R. Embree	1918-1920	Mary E. Ferguson	1932-1951
Roger S. Greene	1920-1927		

DIRECTORS OR ACTING DIRECTORS

Franklin C. McLean	1916-1920	Roger S. Greene	1929-1934
Richard M. Pearce (pro tem)	1920-1921	J. Heng Liu	1929-1938
Henry S. Houghton	1921-1928, 1937-1946	C. U. Lee	1947-

MEMBERS OF FACULTIES AND STAFF

1918-1942, 1947-

MEDICAL COLLEGE

Name	Department	Final Rank	Total Years of Service
Adolph, William H.	Biochemistry	Professor and Head	1948-1950
Alloway, James L.	Medicine	Assistant Professor	1926-1927, 1935-1939
Amoss, Harold L.	Medicine	Visiting Professor	1931
Anderson, Bert G.	Oral Surgery	Assistant Professor	1922-1929
Anderson, Hamilton H.	Pharmacology	Professor and Head	1940-1942
Berglund, Hilding	Medicine	Visiting Professor	1928-1929
Bien, Wan-nien	Medicine	Assistant Professor	1930-1942
Black, Arthur P.	Pediatrics	Associate Professor and Head	1931-1936
Black, Davidson	Anatomy	Professor	1919-1934
Boots, John L.	Dental Surgery	Associate Professor	1939-1942
Branch, J. R. Bromwell	Surgery	Associate Professor	1927-1928
Brackett, E. G.	Orthopedic Surgery	Visiting Professor	1922
Burch, Frank E.	Ophthalmology	Visiting Professor	1940
Cannon, Walter B.	Physiology	Visiting Professor	1935
Carlson, A. J.	Physiology	Visiting Professor	1935
Carruthers, Albert	Biochemistry	Associate Professor	1927-1935
Cash, James R.	Pathology	Professor and Head	1924-1931
Chang, Chi-cheng	Surgery	Assistant Professor	1931-1941
Chang, Ch'ing-sung	Otolaryngology	Assistant Professor	1932-1942
Chang, Chu-pin	Radiology	Assistant Professor	1931-1942
Chang, Chun	Anatomy	Professor and Head	1948-
Chang, Hsi-chun	Physiology	Professor and Head	1927-1942, 1948-
Chang, Hsiao-ch'ien	Medicine	Professor and Head	1924-1937, 1948-
Chang, Hsien-lin	Surgery	Assistant Professor	1929-1942
Chang, Nai-ch'u	Bacteriology	Assistant Professor	1940-1942, 1948-
Chang, Tso-kan	Anatomy	Assistant Professor	1948-
Char, George Y.	Urology	Professor	1920-1942
Cheer, Sheo-nan	Medicine	Assistant Professor	1922-1932
Ch'en, Chih-ch'ien	Public Health	Associate Professor	1932-1938
Ch'en, Graham	Pharmacology	Assistant Professor	1932-1939
Ch'en, T'ung-tou	Biochemistry	Assistant Professor	1927-1942
Ch'in, Kuang-yu	Pathology	Assistant Professor	1930-1942

Name	Department	Final Rank	Total Years of Service
Chin, Yin-chang	Pharmacology	Assistant Professor	1950-
Ch'iu, Tsu-yuan	Public Health	Associate Professor	1931-1942, 1949-
Chou, Chi-yuan	Biochemistry	Assistant Professor	1934-1942
Chou, Chin-huang	Pharmacology	Associate Professor	1949-
Chou, Tsan-quo	Pharmacology	Assistant Professor	1925-1932
Chow, Bacon F.	Biochemistry	Associate Professor	1934-1938
Chow, Hua-k'ang	Pediatrics	Assistant Professor	1940-1942, 1949-
Chu, Fu-t'ang	Pediatrics	Associate Professor	1927-1942, 1950-
Chu, Hsien-i	Medicine	Professor	1930-1942, 1948-
Chu, Kuei-ch'ing (Irving)	Medicine	Assistant Professor	1949-
Chung, Huei-lan	Medicine	Assistant Professor	1929-1942
Cohn, Alfred E.	Medicine	Visiting Professor	1924-1925
Congdon, Edgar D.	Anatomy	Associate Professor	1922-1926
Cort, William W.	Parasitology	Visiting Professor	1923-1924
Councilman, William T.	Pathology	Visiting Professor	1923-1924
Cowdry, Edmund V.	Anatomy	Professor and Head	1918-1921
Cruickshank, Ernest W. H.	Physiology	Associate Professor and Head	1920-1926
Cutler, Max	Surgery	Visiting Professor	1937
Dai, Bingham	Psychiatry	Assistant Professor	1936-1939
De Vries, Ernst	Neurology	Associate Professor	1925-1933
Dieuaide, Francis R.	Medicine	Professor and Head	1924-1938
Dudley, E. C.	Obstetrics & Gynecology	Visiting Professor	1922
Dunlap, A. M.	Otolaryngology	Professor and Head	1918-1930
Eastman, Nicholson J.	Obstetrics & Gynecology	Professor and Head	1924-1929, 1933-1935
Edsall, David L.	Medicine	Visiting Professor	1926-1927
Fan, Ch'uan	Pediatrics	Assistant Professor	1931-1942
Fang, I-chi	Public Health	Assistant Professor	1927-1934
Faust, Ernest C.	Parasitology	Associate Professor	1919-1929
Feng, Lan-chou	Parasitology	Associate Professor	1929-1942, 1947-
Feng, Te-p'ei	Physiology	Associate Professor	1934-1942
Feng, Ying-k'un	Neurology & Psychiatry	Assistant Professor	1936-1938, 1949-

Name	Department	Final Rank	Total Years of Service
Forkner, Claude E.	Medicine	Associate Professor	1932-1936
Fortuyn, A. B. D.	Anatomy	Professor and Head	1925-1942
Frazier, Charles H.	Surgery	Visiting Professor	1926
Frazier, Chester N.	Dermatology & Syphilology	Professor and Head	1922-1942
Fuchs, A.	Ophthalmology	Visiting Professor	1923-1924
Fuchs, E.	Ophthalmology	Visiting Professor	1922
Grant, John B.	Public Health	Professor and Head	1921-1934
Guy, Ruth A.	Pediatrics	Assistant Professor	1924-1929
Hall, Giles A. M.	Medicine	Assistant Professor	1923-1938
Hannon, R. Roger	Medicine	Associate Professor	1930-1934
Harrop, George	Medicine	Associate Professor	1923-1924
Hastings, A. Baird	Medicine	Visiting Professor	1930-1931
Hill, Theron S.	Neurology & Psychiatry	Associate Professor and Head	1937-1942
Ho, Eutrope A.	Public Health	Assistant Professor	1937-1942, 1949-
Hodges, Paul C.	Roentgenology	Professor and Head	1919-1928
Hoeppli, Reinhard J. C.	Parasitology	Professor and Head	1929-1942, 1946-1952
Holman, Emile F.	Surgery	Visiting Professor	1930-1931
Holt, L. Emmett	Pediatrics	Visiting Professor	1923-1924
		(Died in Peking Jan. 5, 1924)	
Howard, Harvey J.	Ophthalmology	Professor and Head	1918-1927
Hsieh, Chih-kuang	Radiology	Professor and Head	1922-1942, 1948
Hsu, Chien-liang	Radiology	Associate Professor	1932-1942, 1949-1950
Hsu, Hai-ch'ao	Radiology	Assistant Professor	1948-
Hsu, Yin-hsiang	Otolaryngology	Associate Professor	1950-
Hsu, Ying-k'uei	Neurology & Psychiatry	Associate Professor	1934-1942, 1949-
Hu, Cheng-hsiang	Pathology	Professor and Head	1924-1942, 1947-
Hu, Ch'uan-k'uei	Dermatology & Syphilology	Assistant Professor	1927-1942
Hunt, Reid	Pharmacology	Visiting Professor	1923
Kappers, C. U. Ariens	Anatomy	Visiting Professor	1923-1924
Keefer, Chester S.	Medicine	Associate Professor	1928-1930
Keim, Harther L.	Dermatology	Associate Professor	1926-1927
Khaw, Oo-kek	Parasitology & Public Health	Associate Professor	1928-1942

Name	Department	Final Rank	Total Years of Service
Kimm, Hyen-taik	Surgery	Assistant Professor	1931-1942
King, Tze	Otolaryngology	Assistant Professor	1921-1940
Korns, John H.	Medicine	Associate Professor	1916-1928
Kronfeld, Peter C.	Ophthalmology	Professor and Head	1933-1939
Kurotchkin, Timothy J.	Bacteriology	Assistant Professor	1927-1940
Kwan, Sung-tao	Surgery	Associate Professor	1924-1942
Leach, Charles N.	Public Health	Visiting Professor	1934-1937
Lee, Chung-en	Medicine Administration	Associate Professor Director	1923-1937, 1947-
Li, Hung-chiung	Dermatology & Syphilology	Associate Professor	1933-1942, 1950-
Li, K'eh-hung	Public Health Hospital Administration	Associate Professor Superintendent	1933-1942 1947-
Li, Ming-hsin	Physiology	Assistant Professor	1949-
Li, T'ing-an	Public Health	Assistant Professor	1926-1934
Li, Tsing-meu	Ophthalmology	Associate Professor	1917-1927
Lim, Chong-eang	Bacteriology	Professor and Head	1922-1942
Lim, Kha-t'i	Obstetrics & Gynecology	Professor and Head	1929-1942, 1948-
Lim, Robert Kho-seng	Physiology	Professor and Head	1924-1938
Lin, Ching-k'uei	Ophthalmology	Assistant Professor	1931-1942
Lin, Sung	Obstetrics & Gynecology	Assistant Professor	1932-1942
Ling, Schmorl M.	Physiology	Assistant Professor	1925-1937
Liu, Jui-heng	Surgery Administration	Associate Professor Superintendent of Hospital Director	1918-1924 1924-1934 1929-1938
Liu, Jui-hua	Otolaryngology	Professor and Head	1919-1942
Liu, Shih-hao	Medicine	Professor	1925-1942, 1949-
Liu, Szu-chih	Biochemistry	Associate Professor	1929-1942
Liu, Yong	Pathology	Assistant Professor	1929-1942, 1949-
Loucks, Harold H.	Surgery	Professor and Head	1922-1942, 1948-1950
Luo, Tsung-hsien	Ophthalmology	Assistant Professor	1932-1942
Lyman, Richard S.	Neurology & Psychiatry	Professor and Head	1932-1937
Ma, Wen-chao	Anatomy	Associate Professor	1921-1942

Name	*Department*	*Final Rank*	*Total Years of Service*
Macallum, A. B.	Pharmacology, Physiology, & Physiological Chemistry	Visiting Professor	1921-1922
Mao, Hsueh-chuin	Dental Hygiene	Assistant Professor	1930-1942
Marlow, Arthur	Medicine	Assistant Professor	1932-1935
Maxwell, J. Preston	Obstetrics & Gynecology	Professor and Head Professor Emeritus	1919-1936 1936-1961
McIntosh, John F.	Medicine	Associate Professor	1928-1932
McKelvey, John L.	Obstetrics & Gynecology	Professor and Head	1934-1938
McKhann, Charles F.	Pediatrics	Visiting Professor	1935
McLean, Franklin C.	Medicine	Professor and Head Director	1918-1923 1918-1921
McQuarrie, Irvine	Pediatrics	Visiting Professor	1939-1940
Meleney, Frank L.	Surgery	Associate Professor	1920-1925
Meleney, Henry E.	Medicine	Associate Professor	1920-1927
Meng, Chi-mao	Orthopedic Surgery	Associate Professor Clinical Professor	1926-1942 1949-
Mills, Clarence A.	Medicine	Associate Professor	1926-1928
Mills, Ralph G.	Pathology	Professor and Head	1920-1924
Miltner, Leo J.	Orthopedic Surgery	Associate Professor	1930-1938
Montelius, George	Dental Surgery	Associate Professor	1929-1932
Mu, Jui-wu	Dermatology & Syphilology	Assistant Professor	1925-1939
Necheles, Heinrich	Physiology	Associate Professor	1924-1932
Nurnberger, Carl E.	Radiology	Assistant Professor	1935-1938
Opie, Eugene L.	Pathology	Visiting Professor	1938-1939
Peabody, Francis W.	Medicine	Visiting Professor	1921-1922
Pearce, Louise	Syphilology	Visiting Professor	1931-1932
Pi, Hua-teh	Ophthalmology	Assistant Professor	1921-1939
Pillat, Arnold	Ophthalmology	Professor and Head	1928-1930, 1931-1933
Read, Bernard E.	Pharmacology	Professor and Head	1918-1932
Reid, Mont R.	Surgery	Visiting Professor	1925-1926
Reimann, Hobart A.	Medicine	Associate Professor	1927-1929
Robertson, Oswald H.	Medicine	Professor and Head	1919-1926
Robinson, G. Canby	Medicine	Visiting Professor	1935
Sallmann, Ludwig	Ophthalmology	Associate Professor	1930-1931
Seem, Ralph B.	Hospital Administration	Visiting Professor	1921-1922
Shen, Tsun-chee	Physiology	Associate Professor	1921-1939

Name	*Department*	*Final Rank*	*Total Years of Service*
Shih, Hsi-en	Urology	Assistant Professor	1929-1937
Sia, Richard Ho-p'ing	Medicine	Associate Professor	1919-1939
Slack, Harry R., Jr.	Otolaryngology	Visiting Professor	1922-1923
Snapper, Isidore	Medicine	Professor and Head	1938-1942
Soudakoff, Peter S.	Ophthalmology	Associate Professor	1924-1940
Spies, John W.	Surgery	Associate Professor	1931-1935
Stevenson, Paul H.	Anatomy	Associate Professor	1920-1941
Taylor, Adrian S.	Surgery	Professor and Head	1918-1927
Ten Broeck, Carl	Pathology	Professor and Head	1920-1927
Teng, Chia-tung	Medicine	Associate Professor	1933-1942, 1948-
Tsang, Yu-chuan	Anatomy	Assistant Professor	1941-1942, 1948-
Tseng, Hsien-chiu	Surgery	Assistant Professor	1940-1942, 1948-
Tso, Ernest S. C.	Pediatrics	Assistant Professor	1921-1931
Tung, Chen-lang	Medicine	Assistant Professor	1924-1941
Van Allen, Chester M.	Surgery	Professor	1930-1935
Van Dyke, Harry B.	Pharmacology	Professor	1932-1938
Van Gorder, George W.	Surgery	Associate Professor	1920-1929
Van Slyke, Donald D.	Physiological Chemistry	Visiting Professor	1922-1923
Wang, Kuo-chen	Medicine	Assistant Professor	1929-1942
Wang, Shao-hsun	Radiology	Assistant Professor	1933-1942
Wang, Shu-hsien	Medicine	Assistant Professor	1930-1942
Wang, Ta-t'ung	Surgery	Assistant Professor	1928-1939
Wang, Yu	Biochemistry	Assistant Professor	1939-1942
Webster, Jerome P.	Surgery	Associate Professor	1921-1926
Weech, A. Ashley	Pediatrics	Associate Professor	1928-1930
Wei, Yu-lin	Neurology	Assistant Professor	1924-1942
Weidenreich, Franz	Anatomy	Visiting Professor	1935-1942
Wen, I-ch'uan	Anatomy	Assistant Professor	1929-1938
Whitacre, Frank E.	Obstetrics & Gynecology	Professor and Head	1939-1942
Willner, Otto	Medicine	Assistant Professor	1920-1929
Wong, Amos	Obstetrics & Gynecology	Assistant Professor	1924-1934
Woo, Shu-tai T.	Medicine	Assistant Professor	1922-1931
Wood-Jones, Frederick	Anatomy	Visiting Professor	1932-1933
Woods, Andrew H.	Neurology	Professor and Head	1919-1928
Wu, Ch'ao-jen	Medicine Public Health	Associate Professor	1928-1939

Name	Department	Final Rank	Total Years of Service
Wu, Ching	Radiology	Assistant Professor	1926-1936
Wu, Hsien	Biochemistry	Professor and Head	1920-1942
Wu, Patrick P. T.	Surgery	Assistant Professor	1935-1941
Wu, Ying-k'ai	Surgery	Associate Professor	1933-1942, 1948-
Yen, Ch'un-hui	Bacteriology	Assistant Professor	1932-1942
Young, Charles W.	Medicine	Associate Professor	1917-1928
Yu, Sung-t'ing	Surgery	Assistant Professor	1939-1942, 1949-
Yuan, I-chin	Public Health	Professor and Head	1927-1942
Zia, Samuel H.	Bacteriology	Professor and Head	1926-1942, 1948-
Zinninger, Max M.	Surgery	Professor and Head	1928-1930
Zinsser, Hans	Bacteriology	Visiting Professor	1938

SCHOOL OF NURSING

The first group of nurses to go to Peking in 1919 with Miss Anna D. Wolf, when she went out as Superintendent of Nurses to organize the Nurses Training School as well as the nursing service of the Hospital, were appointed "graduate nurses" in line with the nomenclature of that period. While the new hospital buildings were under construction, they studied Chinese and served wherever needed in the old Hsin Kai Lu Hospital. By the time the first nursing students had completed a year in the basic sciences at the Premedical School, these nurses were in charge of the new hospital wards where the students received practical training under their supervision and instruction. It was not until 1930 when Miss Gertrude E. Hodgman was appointed Dean that teaching function was differentiated from nursing service, an outgrowth of developments following the *Goldmark Report* of 1924 which had so important an influence on nursing and nursing education in the United States. Even then, academic titles in nursing did not yet connote the degree of competence and experience of the holders as they did in medical schools.

The following list of nurses who participated in the educational program does not attempt, therefore, to give titles or even fields of instruction which changed not infrequently to meet developing needs.

Name	Years of Service	Name	Years of Service
Abbott, Lucy	1920-1923	Dilworth, Jessie	1925-1927
Banfield, Gertrude S.	1921-1924	Downs, Ida M.	1924-1928
Beaty, Mary Louise	1919-1924	Ellis, Ruth	1930-1934
Beaumont, Doris	1930-1936	Filandino, Elvira	1923-1927
Blake, Florence G.	1936-1939	Godard, Winifred	1923-1928
Bray, Linda	1924-1926	Goforth, Helen R.	1920-1922
Brown, Florence	1919-1920	Goodman, Florence K.	1919-1923
Caulfield, Kathleen	1919-1924	Gorey, Margaret M.	1929-1932
Ch'en, Ch'i	1931-1935, 1939-1941, 1947-1949	Grayson, Mary L.	1920-1921
		Griswold, Laura	1924-1927
Ch'en, Lu-teh	1938-1942	Hackett, Elsie M.	1921-1922
Ch'en, Chun-hua	1934-1936, 1949-?	Hall, Frances S.	1920-1921
Ch'en, Shih-feng	1939-1942	Harrell, Virginia	1920-1926
Ch'en, Shu-chieh	1949- ?	Hirst, Elizabeth R.	1928-1937
Chiang, Tsun-chun (Florence)	1940-1942	(Hospital Housekeeping Service, 1937-1942, 1945-1950)	
Chien, Chieh-hua	1935-1942	Hodgman, Gertrude E.	1930-1940
Chiu, Ding Ying	1923-1931	(Dean, 1930-1940; Superintendent of Nurses, 1930-1938)	
Chou, Mei-yu	1930-1931		
Chu, Pi-hui	1926-1932	Holes, Clara A.	1930-1932
Colver, Armeda	1923-1928	Holland, Gladys Lemon	1924-1928
Dalrymple, Lila M.	1921-1928, 1933-1938	Holland, Helen M.	1920-1921
		(Hospital Anesthetist, 1921-1940)	

244

Name	Years of Service	Name	Years of Service
Hsia, Teh-chen	1933-1934	Mooney, Mabel	1921-1925
Hsieh, Louise Tuttle	1930-1940	Mooney, Winifred	1920-1924
Hsu, Ai-chu	1929-1935	Moser, Elizabeth	1935-1938
Hsu, Yu-yung	1933-1940, 1946-?	Moylan, Mary B.	1931-1933
Hsueh, Yi	1929-1935	Moy-Orne, Pearl	1921-1924
Hu, Tun-wu	1930-1933	Muller, Louise M.	1928-1930
Huang, Wu-ch'iung	1948-?	Nieh, Yu-chan (Vera)	1927-?
Hull, Dorothy D.	1933-1936	(Dean, 1940-?)	
Ingram, Ruth	1918-1929	Norelius, Jessie	1928-1929
(Superintendent of Nurses, 1925-1928; Dean, 1925-1929)		Packer, Sophie	1919-1922
		Pai, Hsiu-lan	1917-1923
Jacobus, Dorothy	1920-1923	Pao, Ai-ching	1929-1935
Jen, Hsing-kuo	1921-1938	Parson, Maude	1932-1934
Josselyn, Marjorie	1925-1927	Petchner, Miriam	1938-1940
Kao, Yu-hwa	1924-1938	Polanska, Zenaida	1931-1933
King, Lucile G.	1924-1928	Purcell, Mary S.	1920-1929
Kunkel, Ruth H.	1930-1938	(Superintendent of Nurses, 1928-1929)	
Kuo, Jung-hsun	1927-1938		
Last, Ruth M.	1934-1937	Rinell, Edith	1923-1927
Latimer, Helen F.	1925-1930	Rinell, Margaret	1923-1925
Leach, Glyde M.	1930-1939	Ritchie, Mary A.	1931-1934
Li, Han-ch'iang	1948-1949	Robinson, Ethel E.	1920-1942
Li, Mei-li	1947-1949	Rogers, Grace	1920-1922
Li, Yi-hsiu	1948-?	Schaur, Martha	1919-1920
Liu, Chieh-lan (Belle)	1935-1942, 1948-1950	Scott, Mary B.	1926-1929
		Shao, Kuei-ying	1927-1942, 1948-?
Liu, Chih-chen	1937-1942	Sheh, Yun-chu	1932-1936
Liu, Ching-ho	1937-1942	Shen, Ch'ang-hui	1947-?
Lo, Kuei-chen	1934-1942, 1947-?	Sia, Ming-be	1936-1942
Lo, Yu-lin	1919-1922, 1929-1942, 1949-?	Sia, Yun-hua(Mary)	1931-1946
		Stiles, Katherine L.	1930-1934
(Supervisor, Surgical Supply Room 1949-)		Sun, Chin-feng	1930-1936
		Sun, Tuan	1928-1933
Loh, Anna	1923-1926	Sung, Pao-ti	1932-1936
Lu, Pao-ch'i	1948-?	Sutton, Bertha L.	1919-1922
Lurton, Corinne G.	1930-1931	Sweet, Lula	1919-1929
MacAlpine, Edith I.	1922-1941	Sze, Li-sing (Elizabeth)	1920-1924
McCabe, Anne	1928-1932	Tai, Zing-ling	1922-1925
McCormick, Mildred	1928-1933	Taylor, Erma B.	1928-1931
McCoy, Mary	1919-1924	(Acting Dean, 1929-1930)	
McIvor, Helen	1922-1926	Tennent, Cornelia	1932-1936
Mitchell, Esther	1923-1925	Tien, Tsai-lee	1926-1933
Moo, Mary Priscilla	1922-1923		

Name	Years of Service	Name	Years of Service
Tom, Mabel E.	1920-1921	Wang, Yi	1949-?
(Hospital Admitting Officer, 1921-1932)		Waung, E-tsung (Elsie)	1925-1932
		Whiteside, Faye	1920-1926, 1930-1942
Ts'ai, Heng-fang	1938-1941, 1947-?		
Tso, Han-yen	1935-1936	(Superintendent of Nurses, 1938-1942)	
Uspensky, Margaret	1937-1941, 1947-?	Wolf, Anna Dryden	1919-1925
Wagner, Belle	1934-1937	(Superintendent of Nurses, 1919-1925; Dean, 1924-1925)	
Wang, Ia-fang (Hilda)	1925-1930		
Wang, Hsiu-ying	1937-?	Wong, Chien-chen	
Wang, Loh-loh	1932-1942, 1943-1947, 1948-?	(Margaret)	1932-1939
		Wyne, Margaret M.	1928-1942
Wang, Mei-ying	1940-1942, 1946-?	Yu, Kheng-eng (Kathleen)	1925-1934
		Zia, Ruth V. M.	1934-1939
Wang, Su-yun	1933-1935		

Note: The question mark indicates staff at the time of the Communist take-over about whose subsequent service information is lacking.

PREMEDICAL SCHOOL

Name	Teaching Field	Years of Service
Boring, Alice M.	Biology	1918-1920
Ch'en, Nelson A.	Biology	1924-1925
Corbett, Charles H.	Physics	1923-1925
Downes, Helen R.	Chemistry	1920-1925
Exner, Frank M.	Physics	1922-1925
Feng, Chih-tung	Chemistry	1917-1923
Goodrich, L. Carrington	English	1917-1918
Hogenauer, Alphonse B.	Modern European Languages	1920-1921
Huang, Hui-kuang	Chemistry	1922-1925
Kessell, John F.	Biology	1923-1925
Kwei, Paul C. T.	Physics	1920-1922
Ma, Ch'i-ming (Kiam)	Chinese	1918-1925
Ma, Ming-hsi	Physics	1919-1920
Packard, Charles W.	Biology	1918-1923
Schmertz, Louis R.	English	1924-1925
Scott, Ewing C.	Chemistry	1920-1925
Sears, Laurence M.	Modern European Languages	1918-1919
Severinghaus, Aura E.	Biology (Dean 1923-1924)	1920-1925
Severinghaus, Leslie R.	Modern European Languages	1922-1925
Stephenson, Bird R.	Physics	1919-1925
Stifler, William Warren	Physics (Dean 1918-1922)	1917-1922
Swanson, W. D.	Modern European Languages	1919-1920
Swede, Allen F.	English	1923-1924
Tang, Ning-kang	Chemistry	1922-1925
Tilly, Emily	Modern European Languages	1924-1925
Tong, Y.T.	Physics	1917-1918
Webster, Lorin	Modern European Languages	1922-1923[*]
Wilson, Kenneth O.	Modern European Languages	1923-1924
Wilson, Stanley D.	Chemistry (Dean 1922-23, 1924-25)	1917-1925
Wolf, Edna M.	Biology	1920-1925
Yang, David Kinn	Physics	1922-1925
Yu, C. M.	Chinese	1919-1925
Yu, I. F.	Chemistry	1921-1925
Zucker, Adolf Eduard	Modern European Languages	1918-1922

[*] Died in Peking, July 5, 1923.

ADMINISTRATIVE OFFICERS

Name	Final Title	Years of Service
Alston, William	Chief Engineer	1929-1942
Baker, Dwight C.	Director of Religious Work	1918-1919
Baxter, Donald E.	Business Manager (Hospital)	1918-1922
Bowen, Trevor	Controller (Treasurer 1948-1949)	1935-1949
Bradfield, Vergil F.	Treasurer (Comptroller 1926-1932)	1923-1941
Britland, A. J. B.	Pharmacist	1918-1919
Broomhall, Lyda	Acting Librarian	1922-1923
Cameron, John	Supervisor of the Pharmacy	1921-1940
Chang, C. P. (Archie)	Acting Engineer	1930-1942, 1947-
Campbell, Marguerite E.	Librarian	1923-1927
Chao, T. F.	Acting Librarian	1920-1942, 1948-
Ch'en, James S.	Controller	1925-1942, 1947-
Cook, Mary A.	Librarian	1921-1923
Drummond, Helen Burkett	Dietitian	1934-1940
Evans, Robert K.	Secretary for Religious and Social Work	1922-1923
Ferguson, Mary E.	Chief of College Secretariat	1928-1942, 1947-1950
Gilfillan, Emily	Librarian	1918-1919
Griffiths, Owen A.	Secretary for Religious and Social Work	1939-1942
Hayes, Egbert M.	Secretary for Religious and Social Work	1934-1936
Hogg, James S.	Comptroller	1921-1928
Kiang, V. S.	Chinese Secretary of the College	1929-1942
Li, K'eh-hung	Superintendent of the Hospital	1947-
Liu, Jui-heng	Superintendent of the Hospital	1924-1934
Macmillan, Eva B. A.	Registrar	1922-1928
McCullough, E. Grace	Dietitian	1919-1922
McMillan, Mary	Chief Physiotherapist	1932-1942
Nesbitt, Estelle	Dietitian	1934-1938
Pruitt, Ida	Chief of Social Service	1921-1939
Rugh, Arthur	Secretary for Religious and Social Work	1937-1939
Sloan, T. Dwight	Superintendent of the Hospital	1922-1925
Swartz, Philip A.	Director of Religious and Social Work	1919-1923
Tai, Julie R.	Librarian	1928-1936
Thoma, Katherine	Dietitian	1932-1933
Tsu, Y. Y.	Secretary for Religious and Social Work	1924-1931
Tye, Arthur	Supervisor of the Pharmacy	1932-1942
Wang, S. T.	Superintendent of the Hospital	1934-1942
Wang, Stephen H.H.	Custodian of Clinical Records	1921-1942, 1947-
Wilson, George G.	Supervisor of Buildings and Grounds	1918-1930
Yu, Hsi-hsuan	Chief Dietitian	1935-1942
Yu, Ju-ch'i	Chief of Social Service	1928-1942

REGISTER OF GRADUATES

DOCTORS OF MEDICINE

1924

Hou Hsiang-ch'uan	侯祥川
Liang Pao-ping	梁寶平
Liu Shao-kuang	劉紹光

1925

Liu Shih-hao	劉士豪
Liu Shu-wan	劉書萬
Mu Jui-wu	穆瑞五
P'an Ming-tzu	潘銘紫
Yao Hsun-yuan	姚尋源

1926

Ch'en Hung-ta	陳鴻達
Chia K'uei	賈 魁
Johnson, Hosmer F.	
Lee Shih-wei	李士偉
Li T'ing-an	李廷安
Ling Chih-huan	凌燨桓
Sung Chih-wang	宋志望
Yang Chi-shih	楊濟時

1927

Ch'en Shun-ming	陳舜名
Chu Fu-t'ang	諸福棠
Fang I-chi	方頤積
Fernando, Felino Ch.	
Guna-Tilaka, Yai	
Hu Ch'uan-k'uei	胡傳揆
Ni Yin-yuan	倪飲源
Shen Chi-ying	沈驥英
Wan Fu-en	萬福恩
Yuan I-chin	袁貽瑾

1928

Chang T'ung-ho	張同和
Ch'en Heng-i	陳恒義
Ch'en Pao-shu	陳寶書
Ch'eng Yu-lin	程玉麐
Huang K'e-kang	黃克綱
K'ang Hsi-jung	康錫榮
Li Fang-yung	李方邕
Ling Hsiao-ying	凌筱英
Liu An-ch'ang	柳安昌
T'ang Han-chih	湯漢志
Wang Shih-wei	王世偉
Wang Ta-t'ung	王大同
Wu Ch'ao-jen	吳朝仁
Wu Lieh-chung	吳烈忠

1929

Chang Hsien-lin	張先林
Ch'en Chih-ch'ien	陳志潛
Ch'en Yuan-chueh	陳元覺
Cheng. Jung-pin	鄭榮斌
Chu Chang-keng	朱章賡
Chung Huei-lan	鍾惠蘭
Jung Tu-shan	榮獨山
Li Jui-lin	李瑞麟
Li Wen-e	黎文娥
Lim Kha-t'i	林巧稚
Lin Yuan-ying	林元英
Loo Chih-teh	盧致德
Pai Shih-en	白施恩
Shih Hsi-en	施錫恩
T'ang Tze-kuang	湯澤光
Wang Kuo-cheng	汪國錚

1930

Bien Wan-nien	卞萬年
Chang Mao-lin	張茂林
Ch'en Mei-chen	陳美珍
Ch'in Kuang-yu	秦光煜
Chu Hsien-i	朱憲彝
Chung Shih-fan	鍾世藩
P'an Tso-hsin	潘作新
Wang Shu-hsien	王叔咸

1931

Cha Liang-chung	查良鍾
Chang Chi-cheng	張紀正
Chang Chu-pin	張去病
Cheng Chao-ling	鄭兆齡
Ch'iu Tsu-yuan	裘祖源
Fan Ch'uan	范權
Kimm Hyen-taik	金顯宅
Li, Richard C.	李鉅
Li Wen-ming	李文銘
Lin Ching-k'uei	林景奎
Lu Hung-tien	盧鴻典
Tso Hsueh-yen	左雪顏
Yang Ching-p'o	楊靜波
Yung, Winston W.	容啓榮

1932

Chang Ch'ing-sung	張慶松
Ch'en Hsi-li	陳希禮
Chiang Chao-chu	江兆菊
Chu Mao-ken	朱懋根
Feng Hui-hsi	馮蕙熹
Ho Pi-hui	何碧輝
Hsieh Wen-lien	謝文蓮
Hsu Chien-liang	許建良
Hsu Shih-hsun	許世珣
Hsu Su-en	徐蘇恩

Huang Huai-hsin	黃懷信
Lin Fei-ch'ing	林飛卿
Lin Sung	林崧
Luo Tsung-hsien	羅宗賢
Shih Yung-chen	史永貞
Su Tsu-fei	蘇祖斐
T'ang Jun-teh	湯潤德
Wang P'ei-wo	汪培媧
Yen Ching-ch'ing	嚴鏡淸
Yen Ch'un-hui	顏春輝
Yuan Yin-kuang	袁印光

1933

Ch'en Kuo-chen	陳國楨
Chou Shou-k'ai	周壽愷
Ch'u Ch'eng-fang	瞿承方
Fang Hsien-chih	方先之
Hsu Hsing-an	徐星盦
Hsu Yin-hsiang	徐蔭祥
Huang Chia-ssu	黃家駟
Huang K'eh-wei	黃克維
K'o Ying-k'uei	柯應夔
Li Hung-chiung	李鴻迥
P'eng Tah-mou	彭達謀
Szutu Chan	司徒展
Teng Chia-tung	鄧家棟
Wang Shao-hsun	汪紹訓
Wang Yueh-yun	王耀雲
Wei Shu-chen	魏淑貞
Wu Jui-p'ing	吳瑞萍

1934

Chang Fa-ch'u	張發初
Chao Shu-ying	趙淑英
Chao Yi-ch'eng	趙以成
Ch'en Mei-po	陳梅伯
Ch'eng Yu-ho	程育和
Chou Chin-huang	周金黃

Chou, Willard Y.T.	周裕德
Fan Ch'ang-sung	樊長松
Fan Hai-shan	樊海珊
Fan Jih-hsin	范日新
Hsu Chi-ho	徐繼和
Hsu Ying-k'uei	許英魁
Huang Chen-hsiang	黃禎祥
Ku Yun-yu	谷韞玉
Li Hung-ju	李鴻儒
Ma Yueh-ch'ing	馬月青
Moe, S.P. Paul	墨樹屏
Shen Yu-ch'uan	沈有泉
T'ung Ts'un	童　村
Wang Chi-wu	王季午
Wang K'ai-hsi	汪凱熙
Wu Chi-wen	吳繼文
Wu Shih-doh	吳世鐸
Yang Chien-pang	楊建邦
Yu Huan-wen	俞煥文

1935

Chang, K.P. Stephen	張光璧
Huang, J.J. Theodore	黃仁若
Lin, Hazel	林愛群
Ma, Thomas C.G.	馬家驥
Ma Wan-sen	馬萬森
Su Ch'i-chen	蘇啓楨
Sung Chieh	宋　杰
Ts'ao Sung-nien	曹松年
Wang Shih-chun	王世濬
Yeh Kung-shao	葉恭紹

1936

Ch'en Pen-chen	陳本貞
Chu Wen-ssu	朱文思
Fan Yueh-ch'eng	范樂成
Feng Ying-k'un	馮應琨
Hsiung Ju-ch'eng	熊汝成

Hsu T'ien-lu	許天祿
Huang Ts'ui-mei	黃翠梅
Li Pi-hsia	李壁夏
Liang Ping-yee	梁炳沂
Lu Jui-p'ing	陸瑞蘋
Nieh Chung-en	聶重恩
Wang Hung-wen	王鴻文
Yang Yueh-ying	楊月英
Yu Ts'ai-fan	郁采蘩
Yui, John	余新恩

1937

Ch'en Ching-yun	陳景雲
Chu, Irving	朱貴卿
Feng Yu-shan	馮玉珊
Ho, Eutrope A.	何觀清
Hsu Hsiang-lien	徐湘蓮
Huang Shu-yun	黃叔筠
Ku P'ei-chia	顧培玲
Li Ch'ing-chieh	李慶傑
Liu Gia-chi	劉家琦
Liu Shen-erh	柳愼耳
Liu Wei-t'ung	劉緯通
Lu Kwan-ch'uan	盧觀全
Ouyang, George	歐陽旭明
Pian Hsueh-chien	卞學鑑
Sun Hui-min	孫慧民
Teng Chin-hsien	鄧金鎏
Wen Chung-chieh	文忠傑
Yang Wen-tah	楊文達
Young, Edward	熊榮超

1938

Chang An-lan	章安瀾
Chang E	張　峨
Ch'en Kuo-ch'ing	陳國清
Ch'en Te-lin	陳得林
Ch'en Wu-ming	陳務民

Cheng Te-yueh	鄭德悅	Yu Ai-feng	俞靄峰
Cheu, Stephen Hay	趙伯喜	Yu Sung-t'ing	虞頌庭
Chia Wei-lien	賈偉廉		
Chou, Edward C.H.	周金華		
Chu I-tah	朱義達	**1940**	
Fang Lien-yu	方連瑜	Chang Hsiao-lou	張曉樓
Hsieh Wei-ming	謝維銘	Chang Nai-chu	張乃初
Hsu Hwei-chuan	許萬娟	Chow Hua-k'ang	周華康
Li Tsung-han	李宗漢	Fan Kuo-sung	范國聲
Liang Shao-chao	梁紹造	Feng Ch'uan-han	馮傳漢
Lin Pi-chin	林必錦	Hsueh Ch'ing-yu	薛慶煜
Liu Ch'ing-tung	劉慶東	Kao Ching-hsing	高景星
Lu Ch'ing-shan	盧青山	Koo Chee-hwa	顧啓華
P'an Shih-yi	潘世儀	Lee Yu-chong, George	李雨蒼
Siao Chi-hoah	蕭起鶴	Li Hui-fang	李慧芳
Szutu Liang	司徒亮	Lin Tsuin-ch'ing	林俊卿
T'an Chung-chang	譚仲彰	Ling Chih-ming	凌熾明
Tu Chih-li	杜持禮	Liu Shao-wu	劉紹武
Wang Hsin-fen	汪心汾	Shen T'ien-chueh	沈天爵
Wong Shi-kwei	王師揆	Su Ying	蘇　英
Wu Fang-chen	伍芳貞	T'ien Yu-tao	田友道
		Tseng Hsien-chiu	曾憲九
		Wang Kuang-ch'ao	王光超
1939		Wang Shih-tsuan	王石泉
Chao Hsi-chih	趙錫祉	Yen Jen-ying	嚴仁英
Ch'en Hsi-mou	陳錫謀	Yoh Tse-fei	郁知非
Ch'en Ming-chai	陳明齋		
Chiang Yu-t'u	蔣豫圖		
Chu Tsung-yao	朱宗堯	**1941**	
Hsu Han-kuang	許漢光	Bock, Rudolph	博儒陀
Kwan Han-p'ing	管漢屏	Chang Hsioh-teh	張學德
Lei Ai-te, Edward	雷愛德	Chang Tien-min	張天民
Li Gi-ming	李季明	Ch'en Kuo-hsi	陳國熙
Ling Yung-tung	林榮東	Ch'en Yu-p'ing	陳有平
Liu Yong	劉　永	Chin, Henry	陳郁顯
Soong Han-ying	宋漢英	Ch'u Hung-han	屈鴻翰
Sun Ming, Franklin	孫　明	Fang Yung-lu	方永祿
T'ang Chwen-seng	湯春生	Han K'ang-ling	韓康玲
Wang Cheng-i	王正儀	Ho T'ien-ch'i	何天騏
Wang Chung-fang	王中方	Hsu Ch'ing-feng	徐慶豐
Wang Jun-t'ien	王潤添		

Hu Mao-hua 胡懋華
Huang Nan 黃　楠
Li Wen-jen 李溫仁
Ma Yung-chiang, Joseph 馬永江
Sung Chih-jen 宋志仁
Sung Lu 宋　魯
Teng Ch'ing-tseng 鄧慶曾
Ts'ai Ju-sheng 蔡如升
Wang Te-yen 王德延

1942

Chang Chih-fen 張茝芬
Chang Hsi-hsien 張希賢
Ch'en Min 陳　敏
Chu Liang-wei 朱亮威
Feng Chih-ying 馮致英
Fu Cheng-k'ai 傅正愷
Hsu Chao-chun 徐兆駿
Huang Kuo-an 黃國安
Huang Ts'ui-t'ing 黃萃庭
K'ang Ying-chu 康映蕖
Ku Yu-chih 谷鈺之
Kuo, Kelly C. 郭嘉理
Li Yueh-lien 李月蓮
Ling Chao-hsiung 凌兆熊
Liu Wen-ch'ing 劉文清
Shih Ch'i-nien 石棨年
Su Yuh-chou 須毓籌
Tseng Chao-i 曾昭懿
Wang Wen-pin 王文彬
Wang Yu-sun 王禹孫
Wu Chieh-p'ing 吳階平

1943*

Chang An 張　安
Ch'en Po-shen 陳伯藩
Ch'en Wen-tseng 陳文珍
Ch'en Yueh-han 陳耀翰
Chin K'uei 金　奎
Chu Hung-yin 朱洪蔭
Chung Yung-ken 鍾榮根
Fan Ch'i 范　琪
Feng Pao-ch'un 馮保群
Hsu Ping-cheng 徐秉正
Huang Tzu-ch'uan 黃梓川
Hwang Wan 黃　宛
K'an Kuan-ch'ing, Kenneth 闞冠卿
Kao Jun-ch'uan 高潤泉
Lee Gwoh-chen 李果珍
Lin Hua-t'ang 林華堂
Lu Wei-shan 陸惟善
Soong Hung-chao 宋鴻釗
T'ao Jung-chin 陶榮錦
Wu T'ien-fu, Laurence 吳天阜
Yeh Hui-fang 葉蕙芳

* Degrees granted post-war after all requirements were satisfied.

GRADUATES IN NURSING

1924

Tseng Hsien-tsang	曾憲章

1925

Kong Kwei-lan	江貴蘭
Perkins, Sara	潘愛蓮
Wang Ia-fang	王雅芳
Waung E-tsung	王意貞
Yu Kheng-eng	余瓊瑛

1926

Chu Pi-hui	朱碧輝
Lindberg, Svea A.	令瑞雅
Lin Sz-sing	林斯馨
Sinhanetra, Civili	沈德馨
Tien Tsai-lee	田粹勵

1927

Ch'ao Hwei-ming	晁誨民
Cheo Chia-ih	周家儀
Liu Su-chun	劉素君
Nieh Yu-chan	聶玉蟾

1928

Chou Ssu-hsien	周思賢
Liu Hsiao-tseng	劉效曾
Sun Tuan	孫端

1929

Chang Fei-ch'eng	章斐成
Hsueh Yi	薛藝
Pao Ai-ching	包艾靖
Shih Hung-yueh	史洪耀
T'ao Hui	陶慧

1930

Chao Nai-hsien	趙迺嫻
Chou Mei-yu	周美玉
Chou Mo-hsi	周默希
Hsu Ai-chu	徐藹諸
Hu Tun-wu	胡惇五
Huang Yu-kun	黃毓坤
Kuan Chung-hua	關重華
Kuan Pao-chen	管葆眞
Sun Ching-feng	孫景峰

1931

Ch'en Ch'i	陳琦
Chu Chih-hao	朱志豪
Liao Yueh-ch'in	廖月琴
Sheh Yun-chu	佘韞珠
Sia Yun-hua	謝蘊華
Sung Pao-ti	宋寶弟
Wang Hsiu-ying	王琇瑛

1932

Chang Fang-hsiu	張芳秀
Chu Shu-yu	曲叔瑜
Kuei Yu-teh	桂裕德
Kung Ti-chen	龔棣珍
Su Shu-yuan	蘇淑媛
Wang Loh-loh	王樂樂
Wang Chien-chen	王劍塵
Wu Shun-ch'ang	吳順昌

1933

Chiang Chao-ai	江兆艾
Hsu Yu-jung	徐有容
Li Hsueh-feng	李雪峰
Shih Mei-ying	施美英

1934

Chao Jung-en　趙榮恩
Chen Chun-hua　陳俊華
Chiang Tsun-chun　江尊群
Kuo P'ei-ch'eng　郭佩誠
Lewis, Anna Mae　劉安梅
Liu Chieh-lan　劉潔蘭
Lo Kuei-chen　羅桂珍
Lu Ch'i-ying　盧祺英
Wei Wen-chen　魏文貞
Zia, Ruth V.M.　謝文梅

1935

Chang Hsiu-chen　張琇軫
Ch'en Liang-ch'iung　陳良瓊
Ch'en P'ei-t'ao　陳佩桃
Chu Lien-ch'ing　朱蓮卿
Hsiung Ai-hua　熊愛華
Huang Chih-wei　黃智偉
Li Chia-teh　黎嘉德
Li Huai-ch'in　李懷芹
Li Kuei-chen　李閨貞
P'an Chin　潘　瑾
Ts'ao Hui-chen　曹惠貞
Tso Han-yen　左漢顏
Wang Su-ch'in　王素琴
Wang Su-jen　王素仁

1936

Chan Pao-chiu　詹寶球
Ch'en Liang-yu　陳良玉
Ch'en T'i-yun　陳悌雲
Chou Miao-ling　周妙玲
Ho Chu-hsuan　何祝萱
Huang Min-shan　黃敏嬋
Li Shun-sheng　李順生
Liu Chih-chen　劉志貞

Liu Ching-ho　劉靜和
Sia Ming-be　謝敏秘
Wang Hui-ying　王惠因
Ying Hsi-ying　應惜陰

1937

Chang Yun-fei　張韵斐
Ch'en Jen-ch'ien　陳忍謙
Ch'en Lu-teh　陳路得
Ch'in Yuan-mei　秦源美
Chuan Ju-yu　全如玉
Chu Jui-lin　朱瑞琳
Ho P'ei-fen　何佩芬
Ngai Shih-hua　艾世華
Tuan Yung-chen　段蓉貞
Uspensky, Margaret　吳曼麗
Wen Lu-hsin　文履新
Yu Tao-chen　余道貞

1938

Chang Ts'ai-yu　張才玉
Ch'en Shih-feng　陳士鳳
Ch'en Yu-wen　陳玉文
Cheng Yuan-hua　鄭元華
Chu Pao-t'ien　朱寶鈿
Fei Chiao-yun　費皎雲
Huang Teh-hsing　黃德馨
Ku Hsiu-ling　谷秀玲
Kuo Huan-wei　郭煥煒
Liu P'u-sheng　劉蒲生
Lu Hui-ch'ing　盧惠清
Lu Mei-yin　魯美音
Ts'ai Heng-fang　蔡蘅芳
Wu Yi-sheng　仟儀生
Ts'ao Ching-hua　曹琼華

1939

Ch'en Shao-ch'un	陳少春
Ch'eng Loh-teh	程樂德
Fang Wen-p'ei	方文沛
Huang Pao-chu	黃寶珠
Jen Ch'in-chih	任勤瀞
Ku Ts'ai-kuang	顧彩光
Yang Yu-feng	楊友鳳

1940

Chang Sun-fen	張蓀芬
Chou Hsuan-hsien	周選先
Chou Kuang-tsung	周光宗
Chou Li-pao	周麗寶
Hsu Tzu-mei	徐慈梅
Li Han-ch'iang	李漢強
Li Shih-feng	李式鳳
Liu Chun-tsao	劉滽璪
Shen Shih-hsuan	沈詩萱
Wang Mei-ying	王美英
Wu Chin-yu	吳瑾瑜
Yang Ying-chen	楊英貞
Yuan Yi-chu	袁藝菊

1941

Chang Hui-lan	張惠蘭
Chang P'ing	張 蘋
Chao Mei-te	趙美德
Ch'en Shan-ming	陳善明
Ch'en Yu-chen	陳育珍
Ho Mei-lien	何美蓮
Hsu Pao-ling	許寶玲
Huang Ai-lien	黃愛廉
Huang Meng-ju	黃孟如
Li I-ying	李懿穎
Lin Chu-yin	林菊英
Lin Yu	林 雨

Mei Tsu-yi	梅祖懿
Shen Ch'ang-hui	沈長慧
Ts'ao Fei-hsia	曹霏霞

1942

Chang Te-fen	張德芬
Chang Yun-tsai	張韵菜
Cheng Hui-ya	鄭慧雅
Chiang Tzu-ying	蔣祖英
Chou Jung	周 榮
Chu Chen-mei	朱貞美
Fan Po-sheng	范盇生
Fang Ching-hsuan	方慶萱
Ho Chin-hsin	何錦心
Huang Wu-chung	黃伍瓊
Ku Yung-chen	顧永珍
Li Ching-hua	李景華
Li Mei-li	李美利
Lu Shih-yuan	呂式瑗
Shan Yu-hsin	單又新
Tai Chu-nien	戴祝年
Wu Yun-yu	吳韞玉
Yen Hsiao-mei	嚴筱湄
Yu Fang-lien	于方濂

1943

Chang Shu-chiang	張淑疆
Chang Shu-yi	張淑懿
Li Yi-hsiu	李懿秀
Liu Li-sheng	劉隸生
Lu Pao-ch'i	陸寶祺
Wu Ts'ai-ling	吳采菱

1944

Ch'en Shu-chien	
Ch'ing K'e-hsien	

1945-NONE

1946

Chang Yen-ti	章燕棣
Ch'en Hsing-yun	陳興運
Fei Mei-yun	費美云
Huang Chih-tsung	黃芝聰
Kan Lan-chun	甘蘭君
Li Ch'ung-en	李重恩
Lin Hsiang	林 香
Liu Wang-jung	劉旺英
Shen Wen-yu	沈文郁
Tai Ch'ing-chieh	戴慶捷
Ts'ai Shu-lang	蔡淑郎
Tsang Mei-ling	臧美玲
Wang Han	王 涵
Wang Mei-lin	王美琳
Wu Chen	吳 貞
Wu Ju-ho	吳汝和
Yang Yu-wen	楊玉文
Yu Neng-chih	俞能治

1947

Ts'ao Chu-ping	曹竹平
Wang Shu-ch'in	
Yang P'ei-chen	

1948

Ch'en Shu-chen	
Ch'eng Ch'ung-ch'ing	程崇清
Chou Wen-chih	周文志
Hsiao Chin-ying	蕭金英
Hung Ching-ch'un	洪鏡存
Ma Pi-lien	馬碧蓮
Yang Ying-hua	楊英華

1949

Chang Teh-hsuan
Chao Shih-wen
Ch'en Shan-wen
Chiang Yi-ch'ien
Kuo Chu-fen
Kuo Shu-ju
Li Hsiang-t'ang
Li Hsueh-tseng
Lu Yu-yun
Tsui Ying-jui
Wang P'ei-ch'eng
Wang Yi-chu
Wei Ch'iao-chu

1950

Chang Chi-mei
Chang Yun-hua
Chin Su-hua
Ho Shu-teh
Hsu Hui-hsuan
Hsu Yun-hua
Hu Chu-chen
Kan Lan-ch'un
Ku Cheng-ying
Lin Huang
Pao Teh-chen
P'eng Lu-yun
Ssutu Li-ming
Sung Hsiao-feng
T'ang Shu-lan
Tien Li-li
Tung Chi-fang
Yao Yung-hui
Yen Lo-shen
Yuan Chan-wen

The names in Chinese for some of the post-war graduates are not known in New York.

The Functions of The China Medical Board, Inc., and its relations to the Trustees of the Peking Union Medical College

(Statement approved by CMB November 24, 1936 and by the
PUMC Trustees March 27, 1937)

1. The China Medical Board, Inc., and the Trustees of the Peking Union Medical College are mutually responsible for carrying out the objectives of the Founders of the College as stated by Mr. Rockefeller in 1921 and restated by the China Medical Board, Inc., in 1936.

These objectives include the operation of the Medical College and of its teaching hospital at levels of learning, of teaching, and of institutional stability and influence that will compare favorably with those of leading institutions in other countries, fostering research in the various fields of medicine, providing graduate instruction as well as conducting an undergraduate medical school and school of nursing, and maintaining facilities for the care and study of patients in the several fields of medical practice. These objectives are to be sought with continuing efforts to permeate the scientific and educational program with professional, social, and spiritual idealism.

These objectives specify further that responsibility will be assumed by the Chinese faculty and staff, as individuals are found having maturity, experience, aptitude and character adequate to the discharge of the responsibilities involved.

A further objective is the finding of ways in which, without sacrifice of superior standards, the cost of operation can be kept at a conservative level and brought into reasonable conformity with economic conditions in China.

The China Medical Board, Inc., and the Trustees of the Peking Union Medical College are two distinct bodies, having separate and specific functions, which it is the purpose of this memorandum to define. The joint responsibility is recognized by each board as necessary for the achievement of the foregoing objectives and to that end each board welcomes reciprocal co-operation and advice.

2. The China Medical Board, Inc., is a property-holding body, responsible under its charter for investing its endowment funds and for extending financial support to the Peking Union Medical College and/or other similar institutions in the Far East or in the United States of America. It owns the land, buildings, and equipment of the College, which are leased to its Trustees for a nominal consideration. The China Medical Board, Inc., is obligated by its charter to keep itself currently familiar with the policies, programs and accomplishments of the College, and to review these from time to time in order to evaluate the general trends and quality of performance as related to the objectives of the Founders as stated above. The China Medical Board, Inc., was created for the purpose of furnishing financial support for the furtherance of these objectives as far as the funds available from its own endowments and obtainable by it for this purpose from other sources permit.

The China Medical Board, Inc., stands ready to act as agent in New York for the Trustees of the College, whenever it can be of assistance in matters which are more easily handled there than directly from Peking, and the facilities of its offices are available to the members of the staff and to others sent by the College for foreign study.

The China Medical Board, Inc., or its representatives are ready at any time to advise with the Trustees of the College. To this end the Board endeavors to keep in touch with the general field of medical education, not only in China but also in the United States and Europe.

3. The Trustees of the Peking Union Medical College are responsible for the administration of the College, full powers of initiative and direction being their prerogative and privilege. Their collective judgment on the general principles and procedures most likely to achieve the objectives of the Founders, as restated from time to time by the China Medical Board, Inc., is rendered to the Director of the College, whom they choose and who is responsible to them alone.

The Trustees render annually a full financial report to the China Medical Board, Inc., and submit to it an estimate of the funds required for conducting the College during the following fiscal year. They seek and encourage in China financial support for the College and for associated activities which they may administer.

4. So long as the China Medical Board, Inc., has a director resident in China, he shall serve as the channel of official communication between the two Boards. He renders reciprocal co-operation and advice, welcomed by the two Boards, and participates in adjusting the operation of the PUMC to the financial resources available for its support. He also serves as technical expert in medical education and renders advice in this field to the Trustees of the College, when requested by them to do so.

INDEX

INDEX

wartime activities in Free China, 182-183

China Medical Commissions, First, 18-21, 33, 46; Second, 24-26

Chinese Medical Missionary Association, 19

Chinese National Relief and Rehabilitation Agency, (CNRRA), 203, 205

Chu, Dr.C. K., 127, 132, 183

Chu Fu-t'ang, Dr., 208, 211, 217

Chu, Keats S., 187, 211, 217, 223

Chuan, S. J., 187

Cochrane, Dr. Thomas, 63, 100-102

Coeducation, 38

Cohn, Dr. Alfred E., 114, 123, 145

Committee of Professors, 45, 69, 102, 104, 110, 126, 128, 129

Communists, Chinese, See China

Coolidge, Charles A., 28, 30-34

Cornerstone Laying, 39-40

Cowdry, Dr. E. V., 46

D

Dashiell, L. M., 77

Debevoise, Thomas M., 77, 187

Dedication Exercises, 46, 50-55, 90, 100

Dieuaide, Dr. F. R., 103, 131

Dudley, Dr. E. C., 47

Dunlap, Dr. A. M., 37, 47, 185, 188, 190, 201

E

Edsall, Dr. David, 79-80

Educational Division,
See Governing Council

Eggleston, Margery K., 64, 65, 69, 73, 74, 77, 100, 104

Eliot, Charles W., 15, 17, 18, 36

Embree, Edwin R., 43, 51-53

Exchange Rates, 52, 66, 68, 69-70, 73-76, 78-79, 83, 154-156, 186, 188, 206, 207

F

Fan, Yuan-lien, Mr., 40

Feng, C. T., 38

Feng Ling Chiao, 37

Ferguson, Mary E., 6-9, 177, 185-186, 188, 191, 192, 195, 215, 216, 217-219, 220

Flexner, Dr. Abraham, 15

Flexner, Dr. Simon, 13, 15, 21, 24, 26, 27, 28, 37, 43-44. 59, 63, 64, 137

Foochow, 19, 158

Forkner, Dr. Claude E., 184

Formosa, 19

Fortuyn, Dr. A. B. D., 131

Fosdick, Raymond B., 5, 8, 13, 59, 77, 79, 80, 81, 87-89, 103, 104, 105, 106-109, 111, 114, 117, 145, 181, 190-192, 194, 195, 197-198, 199, 200, 201, 202, 216

Franklin, James H., 15

Frazier, Dr. Chester N., 181

Fuchs, Dr. Ernst, 47

Fugh, Philip, 179-180

Fu, Tso-yi, Gen., 207-209

G

Gates, Dr. Frederick L., 24, 43

Gates, Frederick T., 13, 14-15, 17-18, 21, 22, 43, 89

Gedney Farms Conference, 43-44

Goodrich, Annie W., 59

Goodrich, Dr. L. Carrington, 9, 38

Goodnow, Pres. Frank T., 21

Governing Council, 121, 133, 155
—Educational Division, 121, 128-129, 130-132, 141, 158, 175-176
—Business Division, 121, 129, 133, 141, 150, 151, 175
—Medical Services Division, 121, 129

Grabau, Dr. A. W., 187-188

Gradual and Orderly Development of a Comprehensive and Efficient System of Medicine in China, 17-18

Grant, Dr. John B., 57-58, 71, 132

Greene, Jerome D., 14-15, 16, 18, 21

Greene, Roger S., 8, 18-20, 21, 24, 28, 29, 30, 32, 35, 36, 37, 38, 41, 43, 44, 48, 54, 61, 62-66, 67-74, 75-81, 82-84, 85, 87-89, 91-102, 102-110, 113, 117, 120, 125, 129, 137, 141, 157

Greene, Mrs. Roger S., 8, 86, 107

Gregg, Dr. Alan, 74-76, 77-82, 83-84, 86, 103, 104, 105, 107, 113, 114, 120, 123, 137, 143, 144-145, 161-162, 166, 170, 196, 197, 199, 202

Griffiths, Rev. O. A., 158

Gumbel, R. W., 104

Gunn, S. M., 74

H

Hamilton, Sinclair, 187

Hankow, 18, 56, 72

Harvard Medical School of China, 14-15, 28, 29

Hawkins, F. H., 66, 92

Hayes, Egbert M., 99, 100, 129

Health Station, First, 58, 202, 204

Heiser, Dr. Victor G., 74

Helmick, Judge Milton J., 110

Henderson, Prof. C. R.

Herod, Wm. Rogers, 205-206, 217

Heydt, C. O., 15

Hinsey, Dr. Joseph C., 7, 217

Hirst, Elizabeth H., 185, 191, 215, 217-219, 220
Hodges, Paul C., 37
Hodgman, Gertrude E., 8, 59, 127, 154
Hoeppli, Dr. R., 131, 169, 179, 181
Hongkong, 18, 138
Houghton, Dr. Henry S., 8, 28, 30, 34, 35, 37, 41, 44, 45, 49, 50, 51, 52, 53, 54, 57, 61, 84, 85, 86, 90, 91, 101, 102-103, 104, 105, 106-116, 120, 126, 127-128, 129, 130, 132-137, 138, 139, 140, 141, 142, 143-144, 145, 146, 147, 148, 149, 150, 151, 153-154, 155, 157-159, 160, 161, 162, 163, 164, 165, 166-167, 172-173, 175, 176, 177, 178-180, 181, 184, 186, 190-191, 193, 200
Houghton Library, Harvard U., 8
Howard, Dr. Harvey J., 37
Hsiang-Ya Medical School, 61, 127
Hu, Dr. C. H., 223
Hunt, Dr. Reid, 47
Hu Shih, Dr., 38, 63, 185, 195, 200, 201, 208, 211
Hussey, Harry H., 32-34

I

Ingram, Ruth, 59

J

Japan, 71-72, 128, 129-130, 132-133, 137-138, 152, 153, 169, 171-173, 174-176, 176-180
Jefferys, Dr. W. H., 15
Johns Hopkins Medical School and Hospital, 25, 33, 47
Judson, Dr. Harry, P., 15, 18, 19, 20, 21, 43

K

Keefer, Dr. Chester S., 190
King, Dr. Gordon, 183
King, Sohtsu, G., 66, 155-156, 161-162, 188
Korean War, 218-219
Korns, Dr. J. H., 46
Kronfeld, Dr. Peter C., 131
Kuomintang, 56, 71, 207-209;
   See Nationalist Government

L

Lambert, Dr. Robert A., 190
Leach, Dr. Charles N., 111
Lee, Dr. C. U., 131, 202-203, 205, 206, 210-211, 212, 213-214, 215, 216, 217, 219-220, 221, 222-225, 226
Lester Institute for Medical Research, 46
Li Ming, 188
Li T'ing-an, Dr., 182, 183, 185
Li Yuan-hung, Vice Pres., 18
Library, 66-67, 180, 181, 182, 203
Lim, Dr. C. E., 94, 129, 130-131, 150-159

Lim, Dr. Robert K. S., 109, 111, 125, 130-131
Lin Hsin-kwei, 133, 188
Lin Sen, 72
Liu, Dr. J. Heng (Liu Jui-heng), 62-64, 71, 103, 107, 111, 143, 183, 185, 188, 190, 195, 201, 211
Lobenstine, Edwin C., 120, 129, 134, 137, 143-144, 145, 146, 148-151, 155-157, 160, 168-169, 170, 172, 186
London Missionary Society, 20, 22, 23, 28, 90, 92, 100-101
London Mission Women's Hospital, 29
Loucks, Dr. Harold H., 8-9, 131, 172, 177, 181, 185, 186, 191, 196, 199, 211-212, 213, 214, 216, 218-220, 221, 225-226.
Luce, Dr. Henry W., 15
Lukouchiao, 129

M

MacArthur, General Douglas, 218
MacCallum, Dr. A. B., 46
McCoy, Dr. Oliver R., 7
McKibbin, George B., 18
McLean, Dr. Franklin C., 8, 27-28, 30, 32, 33, 37-38, 39, 40, 41, 43-44, 46-47, 51, 137
McMillan, Mary, 185
McQuarrie, Dr. Irvine, 153
Ma Kiam, 38
Manila, 19, 182
Mao Tse-tung, 214
Marshall, Gen. George C., 193
Mason, Pres. Max, 70, 74
Matsuhashi, Major, 180
Maxwell, Dr. J. Preston, 98, 109, 116, 125
Medical Missions and the Spirit and Teaching of Jesus, 22, 89
Medicine in China, 19-20
Methodist Sleeper Davis Hospital, 29
Ministry of Education, Nationalist, 62-66, 126, 127-128, 134-135, 139, 142, 183-191, 196
   —Communist, 221, 224
Ministry of Health, Nationalist, 58, 63;
   See National Health Administration
   —Communist, 221-222, 224
Mission Boards and Missionaries, 15, 22-23, 25, 89-90, 101, 189-190
Monroe, Prof. Paul, 16, 64-66, 85
Mott, Dr. John R., 15, 21, 23
Murphy, Starr G., 15, 21, 32
Myers, L. G., 64

N

Nanking, 18, 56-57, 111, 158, 196, 212
National Health Administration, 191;
   See Ministry of Health

Nationalist Government, See China
National Medical College of Shanghai, 37,
  127, 177
Nieh, Vera Yu-chan, 154, 174, 177, 188, 204
Norris, Rt. Rev. F. L., 40
North, Dr. Frank Mason, 27, 63
Nursing, new concepts and standards, 29,
  58, 59

O

Ongley, Dr. Patrick A., 7
Oriental Education Commission, 13

P

Parker, Philo W., 200, 217, 218
Peabody, Dr. Francis W., 18, 19-20, 22, 46
Peace Commission, Executive Headquarters, 193, 202
Pearce, Agnes M., 7, 186, 221
Pearce, Dr. Richard M., 43-44, 44-45, 47-
  50, 51-52, 64-65, 68, 74, 95, 96, 120, 137
Pearl Harbor, 171-173, 174, 186
Pei, Dr. W. C., 84
"Peking Man", 84-85, 179
Peking Union Medical College (PUMC),
  charter of, See University of the State
  of New York; contracts, postwar liquida-
  tion of, 186-187;emergency war meas-
  ures, 52, 66, 68, 69-70, 73-76, 78-79, 83,
  154-156, 186, 188, 206, 207; faculty, de-
  velopment of, 45, 46, 57, 130, 131, 206,
  211; scientific aims, statement of, 43-44;
  See Visiting Professors Program
Pratt, Mrs. Miriam I., 185
Premedical School, 37-39
Pruitt, Ida, 90-91
Pu Yi, Henry, 72
Publications, Bibliography, 112

R

Read, Dr. Bernard E., 46, 57, 188
Reinsch, Dr. Paul S., 39
Religious and Social Work, Department of,
  90-102, 113, 129, 158
Robinson, Ethel E., 185
Robinson, E. R., 156, 167-168, 172
Robinson, Dr. G. Canby, 111, 120, 123, 145
Rockefeller, John D., 13
Rockefeller, John D., Jr., 11, 15-16, 18, 21-
  22, 53, 54, 55, 63-64, 87, 88-89, 89-90,
  93, 95, 96, 99-101, 146-148, 150, 157,
  159-162, 192, 198-200, 223, 227
Rockefeller, John D., 3rd, 68, 69, 70, 73-74,
  77, 80, 89, 101, 102, 103, 104, 120, 134,
  145, 146
Rockefeller Foundation, 7-9, 13, 14, 15, 16,
  17, 18, 19, 20, 21, 22, 23, 30, 31, 33, 34-

37, 59-60, 62, 66-68, 70, 80-81, 84-85, 92,
  93-102, 106, 117, 120, 123-124, 127, 195,
  198-201, 200-202
RF-CMB-PUMC Relations, 47, 48, 59, 79,
  102, 108, 114-115, 126, 144-145, 159,
  190-195, 199, 201
Rockefeller Foundation Commission (1946),
  192, 195, 196-201
Rockefeller Institute for Medical Research,
  13
Rockefeller Sanitary Commission, 14
Roosevelt, Pres. F. D., 172
Rose, Dr. Wickliffe, 15, 22
Rugh, Mr. Arthur, 129

S

St. John's University, 36, 39, 177
Schmidt, Dr. Carl, 57
School of Nursing, 42, 58, 84, 112, 122,
  126-127, 138, 141, 167, 174-175, 183, 187,
  188-189, 204, 221-223
Shanghai, 18, 20, 38, 72, 111, 132, 138, 158,
  196, 112
Shanghai Medical School of the RF, 20,
  33-34, 34-37; See University of the State
  of New York
Shields, Dr. Randolph T., 15
Sino-Japanese War, See Japan
Slack, Dr. Harry R., 47
Smith, Dr. Winford H., 33
Smyly, Dr. J. H., 46
Snapper, Dr. I., 175, 178, 181
Soochow, 18, 158
Soong, Dr. T. V., 190
Speer, Dr. Robert E., 15
Stewart, Walter, Jr., 198-199
Stifler, Dr. W. W., 38
Stuart, Pres. J. L., 153, 175, 178-180
Su Huh (Dr. Hu Shih), 38
Sun, T. A., 178, 188, 193, 211, 217
Sun Fo, 72
Sun, Pang-ts'ao, 221, 222-226
Sun Yat-sen, Dr., 56
Survey Commission and Report, 115-124
Swartz, Rev. Philip A., 90-91
Swatow, 18
Sze, Dr. Sao-ke Alfred, 63, 185, 188, 193,
  194, 195, 200-201

T

Tang Shao-yi, 71
Taylor, Dr. Adrian S., 37
Taylor, Erma B., 59
Teilhard de Chardin, 84
Tenney, Dr. Charles D., 15
Tientsin, 18, 72, 132, 133, 139, 177, 210
Tong, Y. T., 38

PHOTO CREDITS: *opposite p.* 16 *group photograph, Rockefeller Foundation Archives; opposite p.* 65 *John R. Mott, YMCA Historical Library; Paul Monroe, Underwood & Underwood; opposite p.* 104, *John D. Rockefeller, Jr., Raymond B. Fosdick, Rockefeller Foundation Archives; Philo W. Parker, Kaiden Kazanjian; opposite p.* 105 *Dr. Alan Gregg, Rockefeller Foundation Archives; Dr. Harold H. Loucks, Udel Bros.; Dr. C. Sydney Burwell, Harvard Medical School; opposite p.* 214 *Rockefeller Foundation Archives.*